THE HER REMEDIES

Herbal Healing
& Practical Recipes
for Everyday Wellness

Ilaria Grandi

Book design by Ilaria Grandi
Cover design by TheBookslab

First Edition: February 2024

Table of contents

15

Introduction

Welcome to "The Lost Herbal Medicine Book," a comprehensive guide designed to bridge the ancient wisdom of herbal remedies with the modern understanding of natural health. I am Ilaria Grandi, a naturopath from the beautiful and historically rich country of Italy. My journey in the world of natural health and herbal medicine has been both a personal and professional quest, deeply rooted in the lush landscapes and rich herbal traditions of my homeland.

This book is born out of a desire to share the profound and often underappreciated knowledge of herbal medicine. It is crafted not only for those with a budding interest in natural remedies but also for seasoned practitioners seeking to deepen their understanding. The strength of this book lies in its comprehensive approach, which combines practical recipes, detailed information on preparation techniques, and insights into the safe and effective use of herbs.

In the following chapters, you will find a treasure trove of information, from ethical harvesting and gathering practices to the preparation of various herbal remedies like teas, tinctures, salves, and oils. Each recipe and formulation is presented in a way that is easy to understand and apply, ensuring that you can integrate these natural solutions into your daily life with ease and confidence.

One of the unique aspects of this book is its focus on the holistic application of herbal medicine. Understanding that true health encompasses the physical, mental, and emotional spheres, we delve into how herbs can support not just bodily health but also mental and emotional well-being. This holistic approach is reflective of my naturopathic practice, where the interconnectedness of all aspects of health is deeply acknowledged and respected.

Furthermore, "The Lost Herbal Medicine Book" stands out for its dedication to the future of herbal medicine. We explore the latest innovations and research in the field, offering a glimpse into how herbal medicine can continue to evolve and integrate into modern healthcare practices.

As we embark on this journey together through the pages of this book, my hope is that you will find not only valuable information but also inspiration to incorporate the healing power of herbs into your life. Whether you are taking your first steps into the world of herbal medicine or are looking to expand your existing knowledge, this book is designed to be a trusted companion on your path to natural health and wellness.

Overview of herbal medicine's role in modern healthcare

This book, "The Lost Herbal Medicine Book," invites you to explore this intersection, shedding light on how herbal remedies not only complement modern medical practices but also offer a holistic approach to wellness that many find missing in today's healthcare landscape.

Herbal medicine, with its roots deeply entrenched in the earliest human civilizations, has evolved over millennia. It represents a rich tapestry of cultural knowledge and natural wisdom, passed down through generations. In recent years, there's been a significant resurgence of interest in these natural remedies, not just as an alternative to pharmaceuticals, but as a way to harmonize with nature in our quest for health.

This resurgence is more than a trend; it's a response to a growing recognition of the limitations of modern medicine in addressing the complexity of human health. While modern medicine excels in acute care and emergency interventions, its approach to chronic conditions, preventive health, and holistic wellness often leaves much to be desired. Herein lies the strength of herbal medicine – it offers a more comprehensive approach, considering the physical, mental, and emotional aspects of health.

For middle-aged women, particularly those who are well-educated and attentive to sustainability and integrated natural medicine remedies, herbal medicine presents an appealing option. This demographic often finds themselves at the center of family health decisions and are increasingly disillusioned with the one-size-fits-all approach of conventional healthcare. They seek methods that are not only effective but also align with their values of sustainability and holistic well-being.

Herbal medicine's approach to common ailments, whether it's a simple cold or more complex issues like stress management and digestive health, often offers gentle yet effective solutions. These remedies, grounded in centuries of traditional use and increasingly supported by modern research, offer a sense of empowerment. Women in this group appreciate the ability to manage health naturally, using remedies that can be easily integrated into their daily lives.

Moreover, the appeal of herbal medicine extends beyond its effectiveness. There's an intrinsic value in understanding and connecting with the ingredients in your wellness routine. It fosters a deeper connection with nature and an appreciation for the subtle yet potent power of plants. This connection is particularly resonant for those who prioritize sustainability. It's about knowing where your remedies come from, how they are harvested, and understanding their impact on the environment.

The ease of integrating herbal remedies into daily routines is another crucial aspect. Time is a precious commodity, and the ability to quickly prepare effective, natural remedies is highly valued. This book aims to provide easy-to-understand, step-by-step information on preparing these remedies. Whether it's a soothing tea for relaxation or a tincture for immune support, the goal is to make herbal medicine accessible and manageable, even for those with the busiest of schedules.

Another significant aspect of herbal medicine is its role in preventive health. In a healthcare paradigm that often focuses on treating illness rather than preventing it, herbal remedies offer a refreshing change. They provide a way to maintain wellness proactively, rather than reacting to health issues after they arise. This preventative approach is particularly appealing to those who are looking to take charge of their health in a more holistic manner.

Furthermore, the role of herbal medicine in mental and emotional well-being cannot be overstated. In an age where mental health is increasingly coming to the fore of healthcare discussions, herbal remedies offer natural options for managing stress, anxiety, and sleep disorders. This aspect of herbal medicine is especially relevant today, as we navigate the complexities of modern life.

Your unique perspective and journey in herbal medicine

Every practitioner carries a unique story – a personal narrative that shapes their understanding, approach, and relationship with the natural world. My journey into the heart of herbal medicine began not in a classroom or a lab, but in the verdant landscapes of Italy, where the natural world is not just a backdrop to life but a central character in its story.

Growing up in Italy, the interplay between humans and nature was always evident. The rolling hills, diverse flora, and the way the seasons dictated life's rhythms - all these elements fostered a deep respect for the natural world in me. It was here, amidst this natural splendor, that my passion for herbal medicine was ignited. This passion was not just born out of curiosity but also necessity. In a country where traditional knowledge is passed down through generations like a precious heirloom, I quickly learned the value of using what the earth provides to maintain health and wellness.

My journey into herbal medicine was as much a journey into history as it was into health. Italy, with its rich tapestry of history and culture, has always been a fertile ground for the blending of traditional knowledge with modern practices. From the ancient Roman use of herbs in healing baths to the medieval monastic gardens, where monks meticulously cultivated and studied plants, the legacy of herbal medicine in Italy is profound. These historical threads wove together, creating a tapestry that tells a story of resilience, wisdom, and a deep connection to the earth.

As I delved deeper into the study of herbal medicine, I realized that this ancient practice is not just about understanding plants and their uses; it's about understanding people, cultures, and the intricate ways in which we are all connected to the natural world. This realization marked a turning point in my journey. I moved beyond merely learning about herbs to understanding their role in a larger ecological and cultural context. It became clear to me that herbal medicine is not a static body of knowledge but a living, breathing discipline that evolves with our understanding of the world.

In Italy, the use of herbs is not just a practice but a way of life. This philosophy deeply influenced my approach to herbal medicine, encouraging a holistic view. It's not just about treating a symptom but nurturing the whole person - body, mind, and spirit. This holistic approach has been a cornerstone of my practice, and it's what I hope to bring to you through this book.

In "The Lost Herbal Medicine Book," you will not find just a collection of recipes and remedies. What you will find is a synthesis of history, culture, and modern scientific understanding. This book is an invitation to join me on a journey that transcends time and geography. It's an exploration of the ancient wisdom of herbal remedies and how this wisdom can be applied in our modern lives.

The strength of this book lies in its ability to bridge the past with the present. By integrating traditional knowledge with modern science, we can create a more comprehensive understanding of health and wellness. This book is a testament to the power of nature's pharmacy and a guide to harnessing its potential in a way that is respectful, sustainable, and aligned with our contemporary lives.

As we embark on this journey together, my hope is that you will find more than just information within these pages. I hope you discover a new way of seeing the world, a deeper appreciation for the plants that share our planet, and a renewed sense of wonder at the magic that nature holds. This book is not just about learning herbal medicine; it's about experiencing it, about feeling connected to a tradition that spans centuries and continents, and about finding your own place in this ancient and ever-evolving story.

As a woman who has navigated the complex path of balancing professional pursuits with personal passion, I understand the challenges faced by our primary readers – middle-aged women with high education, who are attentive to sustainability and integrated natural medicine remedies. You are often the pillars of your families and communities, juggling multiple roles and responsibilities. This book is designed to offer you practical, easy-to-understand, and comprehensive information, tailored to fit into your busy lives without compromising on quality. The recipes and stratagems provided here are not just about saving time; they're about enriching your life with the healing power of nature in a way that is achievable and sustainable.

chapter 1

Chapter 1: The Foundations of Herbal Medicine

History and resurgence of herbal remedies

This ancient art, which spans across cultures and continents, has shaped the foundation of healthcare for millennia. The story of herbal remedies is a tapestry woven with threads of traditional wisdom, cultural practices, and modern scientific inquiry, offering a fascinating glimpse into the human relationship with nature and health.

The Dawn of Herbal Medicine

The journey of herbal medicine begins in the mists of prehistory. Our ancestors, closely attuned to their environment, recognized the healing powers of plants through observation, trial, and often, error.

These early healers were the original ethnobotanists, intuitively learning which plants could heal wounds, alleviate pain, or cure diseases. This knowledge, precious and hard-earned, was passed down through generations, becoming an integral part of community life.

In every corner of the world, indigenous cultures developed their unique herbal practices. The ancient Egyptians, for example, documented their use of herbs like garlic and juniper for medicinal purposes as early as 1550 BC in the Ebers Papyrus. Similarly, in ancient China, the foundational text of Chinese medicine, "The Huangdi Neijing" (The Yellow Emperor's Classic of Medicine), compiled around 300 BC, detailed the use of numerous herbs. Ayurveda, the traditional system of medicine in India, also has a rich history of using herbs, with texts like the "Charaka Samhita" outlining herbal knowledge that dates back to 500 BC.

The Middle Ages and Renaissance

The Middle Ages saw the monastic gardens of Europe become centers of herbal knowledge. Monks meticulously cultivated, studied, and documented a plethora of medicinal plants. The Renaissance furthered this knowledge, with herbals - detailed books describing the properties and uses of herbs - becoming widely popular. These publications, often illustrated with meticulous care, made herbal knowledge more accessible than ever before.

The Turn to Modern Medicine

The advent of modern medicine in the 19th century, with its focus on synthetic drugs and surgical interventions, led to a decline in the use of herbal remedies in the Western world. This shift was driven by rapid advances in scientific understanding and technology, which promised more immediate and potent remedies than the traditional herbal concoctions.

Resurgence in the 20th and 21st Centuries

However, the 20th and 21st centuries have witnessed a remarkable resurgence of interest in herbal medicine. This revival is fueled by a growing awareness of the limitations and side effects of synthetic drugs, coupled with a desire to return to natural, holistic healing practices. People are increasingly seeking sustainable, integrative approaches to health, recognizing that the wisdom of ancient herbal traditions has much to offer in our modern world.

Integrating Traditional Knowledge with Modern Science

Today, the field of herbal medicine stands at an exciting crossroads, where ancient wisdom meets modern science. Researchers are actively studying the efficacy and mechanisms of various herbs, often finding scientific support for traditional uses. This scientific validation not only enhances our understanding of these plants but also helps integrate herbal medicine more effectively into contemporary healthcare practices.

For instance, the use of St. John's Wort for depression, turmeric for inflammation, and ginger for nausea are now backed by scientific studies, bringing these ancient remedies into the realm of evidence-based medicine. This integration is not without challenges, as it requires a delicate balance between honoring traditional knowledge and applying rigorous scientific methods.

Herbal Medicine in the Modern Healthcare Landscape

In the modern healthcare landscape, herbal medicine is no longer seen as merely an alternative but as a vital component of an integrated approach to health. It complements conventional medicine, offering more personalized, patient-centered treatment options. This approach resonates particularly well with those who seek not only to treat illness but also to maintain wellness and prevent disease.

As we delve deeper into the chapters of this book, we will explore not only the practical applications of herbal remedies but also the profound insights they offer into the human body, health, and the natural world. The story of herbal medicine is ever-evolving, and by embracing both its ancient roots and its modern branches, we can enrich our understanding and practice of this timeless art.

The resurgence of herbal medicine is a testament to the enduring power of nature in our lives. It represents a holistic understanding of health, one that is as relevant today as it was in the days of our ancestors. As we move forward, we carry with us the wisdom of the past, the knowledge of the present, and the promise of a healthier, more balanced future.

Integrating traditional knowledge with modern science

This merging is not just a confluence of ideas but a necessary step in evolving herbal medicine into a practice that is both deeply rooted in history and rigorously validated by scientific research.

The Essence of Traditional Herbal Wisdom

Traditional herbal knowledge, passed down through generations, is the bedrock of natural medicine. This wisdom encompasses not just the knowledge of which herb to use for which ailment, but also an understanding of the delicate balance between humans and nature. In many cultures, herbal medicine is not merely a method of treating illness; it is a way of life, interwoven with spiritual, environmental, and community health.

Historically, traditional healers, often known as herbalists, shamans, or medicine men and women, gained their knowledge through a combination of direct experience, oral traditions, and observation of the natural world. This empirical knowledge, developed over centuries, has guided countless individuals through the healing process using the plants and herbs available in their natural environment.

Bridging the Gap with Modern Science

In contemporary times, the field of herbal medicine has gained substantial interest from the scientific community. This surge in interest is not just a resurgence of ancient practices but a recognition of the potential that these natural remedies hold in addressing modern health challenges.

Modern science, with its rigorous methodologies and advanced technologies, offers a way to validate and understand the mechanisms behind traditional herbal remedies. Through clinical trials, laboratory experiments, and pharmacological studies, researchers are unraveling the complexities of herbal medicine, identifying active compounds in herbs, and understanding their effects on the human body.

Synergy for Comprehensive Healthcare

The synergy of traditional knowledge and modern science in herbal medicine provides a comprehensive approach to healthcare. It allows for a more holistic understanding of health and wellness, recognizing that the effectiveness of herbal remedies is often due to a complex interplay of various compounds rather than a single active ingredient.

This integrated approach also acknowledges the importance of context in the use of herbal remedies. The same herb may work differently in different environmental conditions or cultural contexts. Modern scientific methods can help standardize dosages and preparations, making herbal remedies more accessible and understandable to a wider audience, without losing sight of the traditional contexts in which these remedies were originally used.

Case Studies: Blending Traditions with Science

Consider the example of Echinacea, a herb widely used for its immune-boosting properties. Traditional use of Echinacea was based on observational knowledge passed down by Native American tribes. Modern research has since identified several compounds in Echinacea that stimulate the immune system, providing a scientific basis for its traditional use.

Similarly, the use of Turmeric in Ayurvedic medicine for its anti-inflammatory properties has been a practice for thousands of years in India.

Scientific studies have confirmed that curcumin, a compound found in Turmeric, has potent anti-inflammatory and antioxidant effects, validating its traditional uses.

Challenges and Considerations

While integrating traditional knowledge with modern science offers numerous benefits, it also presents challenges. One significant challenge is the preservation of traditional knowledge in a way that respects the cultures and communities from which it originates. There's a fine balance between harnessing the power of these traditional practices for wider health benefits and ensuring that this is done ethically and sustainably.

Moreover, the standardization required by modern scientific methods can sometimes be at odds with the inherently diverse and personalized nature of traditional herbal medicine. Each individual's reaction to a herb can vary based on a multitude of factors, including age, gender, and environmental influences.

Anecdotes from Science, History, and Literature

It wasn't until the 19th century that scientists isolated salicin, the active compound in willow bark, leading to the development of aspirin, one of the world's most widely used synthetic medications. This discovery elegantly showcases the transition from traditional herbal remedy to a mainstay of modern pharmacology.

Turning to history, the story of the foxglove plant, known scientifically as Digitalis purpurea, is particularly enlightening. Traditional healers in Europe used foxglove for various ailments, but its most powerful effect was on heart conditions, though the precise reasons for its efficacy were unknown. In the late 18th century, the English physician William Withering meticulously documented its use in treating dropsy, a condition we now understand as congestive heart failure. His work laid the foundation for the use of digitalis in modern heart medications, exemplifying the historical journey of an herb into the annals of medical science.

From the pages of literature, one can draw upon the enchanting story of Lavender, celebrated in folklore and literature for its soothing and calming properties. Lavender's use is immortalized in Shakespeare's "The Winter's Tale," where it is lauded for its delightful fragrance and medicinal qualities. Modern research has corroborated its traditional uses, revealing its efficacy in reducing anxiety and improving sleep, thereby bridging the worlds of literary homage and scientific validation.

chapter

2

Chapter 2: Harvesting and Gathering Herbs

Ethical and sustainable gathering practices

As middle-aged women, highly educated and deeply conscious of sustainability and natural medicine, you embody the ideal stewards of this ancient practice. Your approach to harvesting is not merely about collecting plants for use but is an exercise in nurturing a harmonious relationship with the environment.

Harvesting with Intention and Respect

The first step in ethical and sustainable gathering is to approach the task with a sense of reverence and intention. When you step into a meadow, a forest, or even your garden to gather herbs, you are entering a living, breathing world. Each plant, from the towering tree to the humblest weed, plays a role in its ecosystem. As you select herbs for harvesting, do so with respect and gratitude. Acknowledge the life of the plant and its contribution to the environment and your health.

Understanding the Impact of Overharvesting

One of the critical concerns in herbal gathering is the threat of overharvesting. Many herbs, especially those that are slow-growing or rare, are susceptible to being depleted. Overharvesting can lead to a significant imbalance in the ecosystem and, in some cases, can drive species to endangerment. It is our responsibility to understand the growth cycles and prevalence of the herbs we seek. By educating ourselves about these plants, we can make informed decisions about which herbs to harvest and which to leave undisturbed.

Sustainable Harvesting Techniques

Sustainable harvesting is about taking only what you need and doing so in a way that allows the plant population to thrive. One of the key principles is to never harvest more than a small percentage of the plants in a given area. A general guideline is to take no more than one-third of the available plants, although this can vary depending on the species' resilience and growth rate.

Another aspect of sustainable harvesting is the technique. For instance, when harvesting leaves or flowers, clip them in a manner that does not harm the main structure of the plant. If you are harvesting roots, it is often best to take only a portion of the root system, allowing the plant to regenerate. Some herbalists practice seed scattering - collecting seeds from the plants they harvest and spreading them in the area to promote growth in the next season.

Timing and Conditions for Harvesting

The timing of your harvest can significantly impact the quality and potency of the herbs. Most herbs have specific seasons or times of day when their medicinal qualities are at their peak. For instance, many flowers are best harvested in the morning after the dew has evaporated but before the sun is high in the sky. Roots, on the other hand, may be most potent if harvested in the fall when the plant's energy has retreated underground.

Weather conditions also play a crucial role. A dry spell may reduce the potency of certain herbs, while others may thrive in such conditions. Being attuned to these nuances not only enhances the quality of your harvest but deepens your connection to the natural world.

Cultivating a Relationship with the Land

Ethical and sustainable harvesting is not just about the act of gathering herbs; it is about cultivating a relationship with the land. This involves regular visits to the places where you harvest, observing the changes in the landscape, the flora and fauna, and the impact of your harvesting practices. It means being an active participant in the preservation and health of the ecosystem.

Leave No Trace Principles

Incorporating 'Leave No Trace' principles is crucial in herbal gathering. This philosophy emphasizes minimal impact on the environment. When harvesting, ensure that you leave the area as undisturbed as possible. This approach extends beyond the act of harvesting to include how you move through the environment, how you transport the herbs, and even how you dispose of any waste.

Harvesting as a Learning Experience

Each harvesting experience is an opportunity to learn. Pay attention to the subtle signs nature offers - the way certain plants grow in abundance in one area but are sparse in another, the insects and animals that interact with the plants, and the overall health of the ecosystem. This knowledge is invaluable, not just for your practice of herbal medicine but for your broader understanding of the natural world.

Giving Back to Nature

Finally, consider ways to give back to nature. This can be through active conservation efforts, planting native species in your garden, or simply spreading awareness about sustainable practices. Your role as a gatherer of herbs is intrinsically linked to your role as a caretaker of the Earth.

Best seasons and conditions for different herbs

Nature operates on a rhythm, a cycle of growth, fruition, and rest, and each herb sings along to this melody. Knowing when to harvest is not just about picking a date on the calendar; it's about observing and aligning with the subtle cues of nature.

Spring: The Awakening

Spring, the season of awakening and renewal, brings forth the tender, vibrant energy of new growth. It's a time when the earth's energy is rising, making it ideal for harvesting leafy greens and early blooming herbs. Plants like nettle, dandelion, and red clover are at their most potent in this period. Their leaves are tender, rich in nutrients, and full of the fresh energy of the season. This is also the time to gather the young buds and flowers of herbs like calendula and chamomile, which are known for their soothing and healing properties.

Summer: The Time of Full Bloom

As we move into summer, the sun's warmth bathes the earth, bringing many herbs to their full potency. This is the season of abundance, where flowers, leaves, and some early seeds are ready for harvest. Herbs like lavender, rosemary, and thyme, bask in the summer sun, concentrating their aromatic oils and offering their full medicinal strength. The flowers of St. John's Wort and yarrow, flourishing under the long daylight hours, are best harvested now for their maximum therapeutic benefits.

Autumn: The Harvest of Roots and Seeds

Autumn is a time of harvesting and preparing for the quieter months ahead. This season is ideal for gathering roots and seeds, as the plants draw their energy back into the earth. It is the perfect time to unearth roots like echinacea, valerian, and burdock, which have stored a season's worth of nutrients. Seeds like fennel, caraway, and milk thistle, having matured over the summer, are also ready to be collected. These parts of the plant, rich in energy and strength, are potent allies for the winter months.

Winter: The Quiet Collection

Winter, often seen as a time of rest in the plant world, still offers gifts for those who know where to look. Evergreens like pine, fir, and cedar hold their vitality throughout the colder months, offering immune-supporting properties. It's also a time for introspection and planning for the year ahead, identifying which herbs to cultivate and gather in the coming seasons.

Honoring the Conditions: Beyond the Seasons

While seasons play a crucial role in determining the best time to harvest, understanding the specific conditions that each herb thrives in is equally important. This knowledge not only guarantees the quality and efficacy of the herbs but also ensures their sustainable and ethical gathering.

Sun and Shade: The Light Lovers and the Shelter Seekers

Some herbs, like basil and rosemary, revel in the full sun, accumulating their essential oils and medicinal compounds under the bright light. Others, such as lemon balm and mint, prefer the dappled shade, where they retain their delicate flavors and aromas without the stress of direct, scorching sun.

Soil and Moisture: The Earth's Embrace

The nature of the soil and the level of moisture it holds significantly impact the quality of the herbs.

Plants like marshmallow and horsetail, which grow in moist, almost boggy conditions, develop a different profile of compounds compared to those like lavender and thyme, which thrive in dry, well-drained soils. Understanding these preferences helps in both cultivating these herbs in your garden and seeking them out in their natural habitats.

Elevation and Climate: The Highs and Lows

Elevation and the accompanying climate play a critical role in the growth of certain herbs. For instance, mountain herbs like arnica and yarrow, adapted to high altitudes and cooler temperatures, develop robust compounds to protect themselves, which in turn can be beneficial in herbal remedies.

The Art of Observation: Becoming One with Nature

A key aspect of harvesting herbs is developing a keen sense of observation. Watching the cycles of the moon, the patterns of the weather, and the behavior of the plants themselves offers invaluable insights. The best herbalists are those who listen to the whispers of nature, understanding that each plant has its own perfect moment of harvest.

Integrating Harvesting into Busy Lives

For the modern woman, integrating the practice of harvesting herbs can seem like a daunting addition to an already busy schedule. However, it can be seamlessly woven into daily life. Whether it's a weekend foray into the forest, a quiet moment in the garden, or even selecting the right time to gather herbs from your balcony planters, these practices can become meditative, grounding, and deeply rewarding. They offer a connection to the earth and a tangible way to take control of your health and well-being.

chapter

3

Chapter 3: Preparation Techniques for Herbal Remedies

Step-by-step guides for teas, tinctures, salves, and oils

Our focus is on creating teas, tinctures, salves, and oils, each with its unique preparation method and healing properties. These remedies provide a hands-on way to connect with the healing power of nature and offer a rewarding experience in the creation of your own health aids.

Teas: The Art of Infusion and Decoction

Herbal teas, a cornerstone in the world of herbal remedies, are both accessible and profoundly effective. The creation of an herbal tea is an art that involves either infusion or decoction, techniques that differ based on the part of the plant used. While infusion is perfect for harnessing the gentle qualities of leaves and flowers, decoction is tailored to extract the robust properties from roots, barks, and seeds.

Infusion: Unveiling the Delicate Strength of Plants

Infusion is a delicate process, ideal for preserving the subtle yet powerful essences of leaves and flowers. For example, consider making a calming chamomile tea. Start by boiling water. Once it reaches a rolling boil, remove it from heat. Add about one teaspoon of dried chamomile flowers or two teaspoons if you're using fresh flowers, per cup of boiling water. Covering the pot or cup is crucial — it traps the steam and the essential oils that would otherwise evaporate. Let it steep for about 5 to 15 minutes.

The steeping time is important to consider. For instance, steeping chamomile for 5 minutes creates a mild, soothing tea, perfect for a gentle nudge towards relaxation. Extending it to 10 or 15 minutes, however, releases more of its calming properties, making it ideal for pre-bedtime consumption to aid sleep. This method, by not directly boiling the plant material, keeps the delicate oils and flavors intact, offering a tea that is both therapeutic and pleasant to the taste.

Decoction: Extracting Deep-Rooted Benefits

Decoction is a more intensive process, designed to draw out the deeper essences from tougher plant materials like roots, barks, or seeds. For example, when preparing a ginger tea, known for its digestive and anti-inflammatory properties, the decoction method is ideal. Begin by slicing about one inch of fresh ginger root. Place these slices in about two cups of cold water. Slowly bring the water to a boil, and then reduce the heat to let it simmer gently.

The simmering time can range from 20 to 45 minutes. For a milder tea, a 20-minute simmer is sufficient, but for a more potent brew, especially if you're seeking substantial digestive aid or are dealing with severe inflammation, a longer simmer of up to 45 minutes is more effective. This extended simmering time allows the tougher fibers of the ginger root to break down, releasing both its bold flavor and its potent medicinal compounds.

In Practice: Making Your Herbal Tea

Let's bring these concepts to life with a couple of examples. Say you're feeling anxious and need something to calm your nerves. A lemon balm infusion would be your go-to. Take two teaspoons of fresh lemon balm leaves (or one teaspoon if dried) per cup of hot water. Steep it covered for about 10 minutes. The result is a soothing, mildly citrus-flavored tea that eases anxiety and promotes relaxation.

Alternatively, if you're dealing with a stubborn cough and need a strong expectorant, a decoction of licorice root would be beneficial. Use about one teaspoon of chopped licorice root per cup of cold water. Bring it to a boil and then simmer for approximately 30 minutes. This longer simmering time ensures that all the expectorant qualities of the licorice are thoroughly extracted, providing you with a potent remedy for your cough.

Tinctures: Concentrated Herbal Power

Tinctures represent a potent and enduring tradition in herbal medicine. These alcohol-based herbal extracts capture the essence of herbs in a concentrated form, offering a longer shelf life and a more potent dose than their tea counterparts. The creation of a tincture is a meticulous yet rewarding process, involving the extraction of active constituents from herbs into a solvent, typically a blend of alcohol and water.

The Alchemy of Tinctures: The Process Explained

The process of making a tincture starts with the selection and preparation of herbs. For instance, consider creating a tincture from Echinacea, known for its immune-boosting properties. Begin by finely chopping or grinding the Echinacea, whether it's fresh or dried. The finer the herb is chopped, the more surface area is exposed to the solvent, ensuring a more thorough extraction.

Next, choose your solvent. The most common and effective solvent is a mixture of water and alcohol. The alcohol preserves the tincture and extracts a wide range of water-soluble and fat-soluble compounds from the herbs. Vodka, with its neutral flavor and around 40% alcohol content, is a popular choice. For a stronger extraction, brandy, with its slightly higher alcohol content, can be used.

The ratio of herb to solvent is critical. A general guideline is to use one part herb to two parts solvent. This ratio ensures that the solvent is sufficient to extract the active compounds from the herbs effectively. In a clean jar, mix the chopped Echinacea with the vodka or brandy. Ensure that the herbs are completely submerged in the solvent to prevent any spoilage or mold growth.

Steeping and Shaking: The Maturation of a Tincture

Once the herbs and solvent are combined, seal the jar tightly and store it in a cool, dark place. This storage is crucial as light and heat can degrade the tincture. Shaking the jar daily is an essential part of the process. Each shake agitates the mixture, ensuring that the solvent comes into contact with all parts of the herb, thereby optimizing the extraction.

The steeping period for tinctures can vary. Typically, it ranges from two to six weeks. The length of time depends on the herb used and the desired strength of the tincture. For example, a tincture made with Echinacea may be ready in as little as two weeks, but allowing it to steep for four to six weeks will produce a more potent extract.

Straining and Storing: Finalizing Your Tincture

After the steeping period, the next step is to strain the tincture. Pour the mixture through a fine mesh or cheesecloth into another container, squeezing out as much liquid as possible. This straining process removes all solid plant materials, leaving behind the concentrated liquid extract.

The final step is to transfer the tincture into dark glass dropper bottles. The dark glass protects the tincture from light, preserving its potency. Labeling the bottles with the name of the herb and the date of preparation will help you keep track of your tincture's shelf life and contents.

In Practice: Crafting a Tincture for Everyday Use

Let's take the example of creating a valerian root tincture, widely used for its sedative properties. After chopping the valerian root, follow the same process of mixing it with the alcohol-water solvent in the appropriate ratio. After steeping for the recommended period, you'll have a potent tincture that can be used to aid sleep or alleviate anxiety. A standard dose might be a few drops to a full dropper, depending on your needs and the strength of the tincture.

Salves: Healing Ointments for Topical Use

Salves, the soothing balms of herbal medicine, are thickened ointments renowned for their efficacy in treating various skin conditions, healing wounds, and easing muscle aches. These versatile preparations are made by infusing oil with therapeutic herbs and then thickening the mixture with beeswax. The process of making a herbal salve is both an art and a science, offering a deeply satisfying way to create a personalized remedy.

The Infusion: Crafting the Herbal Oil Base

The journey of making a salve begins with the infusion of oil with your chosen herbs. This process extracts the active compounds of the herbs into the oil, creating a potent and therapeutic base. For instance, if you're aiming to create a salve for soothing inflamed skin, calendula is an excellent choice due to its anti-inflammatory properties.

Start by selecting a carrier oil. Common choices include coconut oil, known for its skin-nourishing properties, and olive oil, which is rich in antioxidants. Place your dried calendula petals in a double boiler, and then pour the carrier oil over them, ensuring the petals are fully submerged. The double boiler is essential as it provides gentle, indirect heat, preventing the herbs from frying, which can diminish their medicinal properties.

Gently heat the mixture on low for about three hours. This slow infusion allows for a thorough extraction of the healing compounds from the calendula petals into the oil. It's important to stir occasionally and monitor the heat to maintain a consistent temperature.

Straining and Mixing: From Infused Oil to Salve

Once the oil is richly infused with the calendula's essence, the next step is straining. Line a strainer with cheesecloth and pour the oil mixture through it, collecting the infused oil in a bowl. Squeeze the cheesecloth to extract as much oil as possible from the remaining plant material.

Now, it's time to turn this infused oil into a salve by adding beeswax. The ratio of beeswax to oil is key to achieving the right consistency. Generally, one ounce of beeswax per cup of herbal oil strikes the perfect balance. Grate the beeswax and add it to the infused oil. Gently heat this mixture, stirring occasionally, until the beeswax completely melts and blends with the oil.

Customization: Enhancing Your Salve

At this stage, you have the option to customize your salve. For added therapeutic benefits and fragrance, consider incorporating essential oils. For the calendula salve, lavender or chamomile essential oils can be a great addition for their soothing and anti-inflammatory properties. Add a few drops of essential oil to the melted mixture after removing it from the heat.

Setting and Storing: Final Steps

Pour the finished liquid into small tins or jars. Allow the salve to cool and solidify at room temperature. As it cools, the mixture will transform from a liquid to a semi-solid state, ready for use. Label your salve with the ingredients and date of creation.

In Practice: Creating a Muscle Soothe Salve

Let's illustrate this process with another example. To create a salve for muscle aches, you might choose arnica, known for its pain-relieving properties. Follow the same process of infusing the arnica in oil, straining, and then adding beeswax. For extra pain relief, adding a few drops of peppermint essential oil, which has natural analgesic properties, can enhance the effectiveness of your muscle soothe salve.

Oils: Herbal Infusions for External and Internal Use

Herbal oils, with their multipurpose applications, are a staple in both traditional and contemporary herbal practices. These oils are not just carriers of the healing properties of herbs but also serve as a medium that can be adapted for various uses – from therapeutic massage and skincare to culinary enhancements. The method of preparing an herbal oil is simple yet profound, capturing the essence of herbs in a versatile and accessible form.

The Process of Infusion: Creating Your Herbal Oil

The process of infusing oil with herbs is an exercise in patience and precision. The solar infusion method is a popular and effective technique. To begin, select a herb based on your intended use. For example, St. John's Wort is an excellent choice for a massage oil intended to relieve nerve pain, while rosemary can be infused for a culinary oil.

Fill a clean, dry jar with your chosen dried herb. It's crucial to use dried herbs to prevent moisture from entering the oil, which can lead to spoilage. Cover the herbs completely with a carrier oil. Olive oil is a great all-purpose choice, but for skincare, oils like sweet almond or jojoba can be more suitable due to their lighter texture and skin-nourishing properties.

Once the herbs are submerged in oil, seal the jar tightly. Place it in a sunny window where it will receive ample sunlight. This warmth from the sun gently heats the oil, facilitating the release of active compounds from the herbs into the oil. It's a gentle process that honors the delicate nature of the herbs.

Shake the jar daily. This simple act ensures that all parts of the herbs are in contact with the oil, promoting an even and thorough infusion.

The Duration of Infusion

The length of the infusion process can vary depending on the herb and the desired potency.

Generally, a period of two to four weeks is recommended. For instance, a St. John's Wort oil may reach its optimal potency at around four weeks, while a rosemary culinary oil might be ready in two weeks.

Straining and Storing the Herbal Oil

After the infusion period, it's time to strain the oil. Pour the mixture through a fine mesh or cheesecloth, squeezing to extract as much oil as possible. The resulting herbal oil should be clear and free from plant debris.

Store the strained oil in a cool, dark place. Amber or dark-colored glass bottles are ideal as they protect the oil from light, which can degrade its quality.

Applications of Herbal Oils

Herbal oils can be used in various ways. A St. John's Wort-infused oil, for example, can be applied topically to soothe nerve pain, burns, or wounds. Its anti-inflammatory and analgesic properties make it a valuable addition to any home remedy kit.

In the culinary realm, a rosemary-infused olive oil can elevate simple dishes with its robust flavor. It's perfect for drizzling over roasted vegetables, pasta, or fresh bread.

Further Processing: Transforming Oil into Salves and Creams

Herbal oils can also be a base for creating more complex herbal preparations like salves or creams. For instance, the St. John's Wort oil can be further processed with beeswax to create a soothing salve for topical application.

Tips for ensuring potency and purity

As we delve into this fundamental aspect of preparing herbal remedies, it is vital to understand that the strength and purity of your herbal concoctions are not just by-products of the ingredients you choose; they are the embodiment of the care, attention, and knowledge you put into every step of the process.

Potency in herbal remedies refers to the strength and effectiveness of the active constituents within the herbs. This potency is not static; it varies based on several factors, from the way the herbs are grown and harvested to how they are stored and prepared.

Cultivation and Harvest

The journey to potent herbal remedies begins long before the herbs reach your kitchen or workshop. It starts with how these herbs are cultivated and when they are harvested. Herbs grown in their native environment, where they can thrive without excessive human intervention, often develop a robust profile of active constituents. Organic cultivation methods that shun chemical pesticides and fertilizers contribute significantly to the potency of herbs by ensuring that the plants can channel their energy into developing their natural medicinal qualities.

The timing of the harvest is just as critical. Many herbs reach their peak potency at specific times in their growth cycle. For instance, some herbs are most potent when harvested just before they bloom, as this is when they concentrate their energy and active constituents in the leaves and stems. Understanding these nuances for each herb is crucial for ensuring that you're gathering them at their most potent.

Drying and Storage

Once harvested, how you dry and store herbs plays a pivotal role in preserving their potency. Herbs should be dried slowly, away from direct sunlight, and in an area with good air circulation. This process preserves the delicate oils and active compounds within the herbs. Overheating or prolonged exposure to light can degrade these compounds, diminishing the herb's effectiveness.

Proper storage is equally important. Herbs should be stored in airtight containers, away from light and moisture, which can lead to mold growth and degradation of the herbs. Glass jars with tight-fitting lids are ideal for this purpose. Remember, even the best herbs can lose their potency if not stored correctly.

The Imperative of Purity

Purity in herbal remedies is about ensuring that the herbs and the final product are free from contaminants that could harm your health or dilute the efficacy of the remedy. This purity is not just about the absence of chemical pollutants; it extends to the cleanliness of the herbs and the environment in which they are processed.

Cleanliness of Herbs

Start with clean, high-quality herbs. If you're foraging, be mindful of the environment from which you gather your herbs. Areas away from roads, industrial sites, and agricultural fields that might use pesticides are preferable. If you're purchasing herbs, choose reputable sources that provide organic, ethically-sourced herbs.

Washing herbs might seem like a straightforward task, but it's a critical step in maintaining purity. Rinse herbs under cool, running water to remove any dirt or small insects. For roots, scrubbing might be necessary. After washing, pat them dry gently with a clean cloth or let them air dry.

Processing Environment

The area where you prepare your herbal remedies should be as clean and controlled as possible. Ensure that the surfaces, utensils, and containers you use are clean and free from contaminants. This includes everything from the chopping board and knife to the pots and jars you use for storing your remedies. Cross-contamination can occur easily, so maintaining a clean workspace is paramount for ensuring the purity of your herbal products.

Steeping, Infusing, and Mixing

The actual preparation of the remedy is where your potency and purity efforts come to fruition. Whether you are steeping a tea, infusing oil, or mixing a salve, temperature and time are crucial factors. Heat helps to extract the active compounds from herbs, but too much heat can destroy them. Learn the optimal temperatures and steeping times for each herb to maximize their medicinal properties.

When infusing oils or creating salves, use a double boiler to gently heat the herbs. This indirect heat allows for better control and helps prevent overheating. For teas, boiling water can be too harsh for some delicate herbs. Instead, use hot water that's just below boiling, and steep for the recommended amount of time to extract the beneficial properties effectively.

chapter
4

Chapter 4: Herbal Recipes for Everyday Health

Simple recipes for common ailments (e.g., colds, digestion, stress)

In this chapter, we delve into the heart of herbal medicine: practical, simple, and effective recipes to address common ailments. These recipes are designed to be easy to prepare, using ingredients that are generally safe and widely available. Each recipe will include detailed instructions for preparation, storage, and usage, along with precautions and recommended durations for treatment.

Soothing Chamomile Tea for Stress Relief

Ingredients: Chamomile flowers, hot water

Preparation: Steep 2 teaspoons of dried chamomile flowers in 1 cup of hot water for 5-10 minutes.

Storage: Best consumed fresh; can be refrigerated for

up to 24 hours. **Usage**: Drink 1 cup in the evening or when feeling stressed. **Duration**: Safe for daily use. **Precautions**: Avoid if allergic to ragweed.

Ginger Tea for Digestion

Ingredients: Fresh ginger root, hot water, honey (optional) **Preparation**: Slice 1-2 inches of fresh ginger root and steep in boiling water for 10-15 minutes. Add honey to taste. **Storage**: Best enjoyed fresh; can be stored in the refrigerator for up to 2 days. **Usage**: Drink 1 cup after meals. **Duration**: Suitable for daily use. **Precautions**: May interfere with blood thinners.

Echinacea Tincture for Colds

Ingredients: Echinacea root, vodka **Preparation**: Fill a jar with dried echinacea root and cover with vodka. Seal and store in a cool, dark place for 4-6 weeks, shaking daily. **Storage**: Store in a dark bottle, away from light. Lasts up to 2 years. **Usage**: Take 1-2 ml up to three times daily at the first sign of a cold.

Duration: Not to exceed 10 days. **Precautions**: May interact with immune-suppressing drugs.

Peppermint Oil Rub for Headaches

Ingredients: Peppermint essential oil, carrier oil (like almond or jojoba) **Preparation**: Mix 5 drops of peppermint essential oil with 1 ounce of carrier oil. **Storage**: Store in an airtight container, away from light. **Usage**: Massage a small amount onto temples and forehead. **Duration**: Use as needed. **Precautions**: Avoid contact with eyes.

Lemon Balm Sleepy Time Tea

Ingredients: Lemon balm leaves, hot water **Preparation**: Steep 1 tablespoon of dried lemon balm leaves in 1 cup of hot water for 10 minutes. **Storage**: Best consumed fresh; refrigerate for up to 24 hours. **Usage**: Drink 1 cup 30 minutes before bedtime. **Duration**: Safe for nightly use. **Precautions**: May interact with sedatives.

Turmeric and Honey Paste for Sore Throat

Ingredients: Turmeric powder, honey **Preparation**: Mix 1 teaspoon of turmeric powder with enough honey to form a paste. **Storage**: Use immediately; can be stored in the refrigerator for up to 48 hours. **Usage**: Take ½ teaspoon of the paste and swallow slowly. **Duration**: Use every few hours as needed. **Precautions**: Avoid if allergic to turmeric.

Lavender Essential Oil for Anxiety

Ingredients: Lavender essential oil, diffuser or carrier oil **Preparation**: Use in a diffuser or mix a few drops with a carrier oil for topical application. **Storage**: Keep the essential oil in its original dark glass bottle, away from light. **Usage**: Diffuse in the evening or apply topically when feeling anxious. **Duration**: Use as needed. **Precautions**: Can cause skin irritation if not diluted.

Dandelion Tea for Liver Support

Ingredients: Dandelion leaves or root, hot water **Preparation**: Steep 1-2 teaspoons of dandelion in 1 cup of hot water for 10 minutes. **Storage**: Best consumed fresh; can be stored in the refrigerator for 24 hours. **Usage**: Drink 1 cup daily. **Duration**: Suitable for daily use. **Precautions**: May interact with diuretics.

Nettle Infusion for Allergies

Ingredients: Dried nettle leaves, hot water **Preparation**: Steep 1-2 tablespoons of dried nettle leaves in 1 cup of hot water for 10-15 minutes. **Storage**: Drink fresh; store any leftovers in the refrigerator for up to 24 hours. **Usage**: Drink 1 cup daily during allergy season. **Duration**: Suitable for daily use during allergy season. **Precautions**: May interact with blood pressure medication.

Calendula Salve for Skin Irritations

Ingredients: Calendula flowers, olive oil, beeswax **Preparation**: Infuse olive oil with calendula flowers; strain and mix with melted beeswax to form a salve. **Storage**: Store in a cool, dry place in an airtight container. **Usage**: Apply to affected skin areas as needed. **Duration**: Use as needed. **Precautions**: Patch test for allergic reactions.

Cinnamon and Ginger Warm Tea for Fatigue

Ingredients: Cinnamon stick, fresh ginger root, hot water **Preparation**: Boil a cinnamon stick and a slice of ginger in water for 10 minutes. **Storage**: Best consumed fresh; can be stored in the refrigerator for up to 24 hours. **Usage**: Drink 1 cup in the morning or when feeling fatigued. **Duration**: Safe for daily use. **Precautions**: May interact with blood sugar medication.

Raspberry Leaf Tea for Menstrual Cramps

Ingredients: Dried raspberry leaves, hot water **Preparation**: Steep 1 tablespoon of dried leaves in 1 cup of hot water for 15 minutes. **Storage**: Best consumed fresh; can be refrigerated for up to 48 hours. **Usage**: Drink 1-2 cups daily during menstrual cycle. **Duration**: Use during menstrual periods. **Precautions**: Consult a healthcare provider if pregnant.

Arnica Massage Oil for Muscle Soreness

Ingredients: Arnica flowers, carrier oil (e.g., almond oil) **Preparation**: Infuse arnica flowers in carrier oil for 2-4 weeks; strain. **Storage**: Store in a dark, airtight container away from light. **Usage**: Massage into sore muscles as needed. **Duration**: Use as needed. **Precautions**: For external use only; avoid broken skin.

Willow Bark Tea for Joint Pain

Ingredients: Willow bark, hot water **Preparation**: Steep 1 teaspoon of bark in 1 cup of hot water for 20 minutes. **Storage**: Best consumed fresh; can be refrigerated for up to 24 hours. **Usage**: Drink 1 cup daily. **Duration**: Not to exceed 6 weeks. **Precautions**: Similar to aspirin; avoid if allergic or on blood thinners.

Elderberry Syrup for Immune Boosting

Ingredients: Dried elderberries, water, honey **Preparation**: Simmer elderberries in water, strain, and mix with honey. **Storage**: Store in a refrigerator for up to 2 months. **Usage**: Take 1 tablespoon daily during cold and flu season. **Duration**: Safe for daily use during cold seasons. **Precautions**: Raw elderberries can be toxic; ensure they are properly cooked.

Peppermint and Eucalyptus Bath Soak for Relaxation

Ingredients: Peppermint leaves, eucalyptus leaves, Epsom salt **Preparation**: Mix leaves with Epsom salt; add to a warm bath. **Storage**: Store the dry mix in an airtight container. **Usage**: Use 1 cup in a bath when needed. **Duration**: Use as needed. **Precautions**: Patch test for skin sensitivity.

Hawthorn Berry Tonic for Heart Health

Ingredients: Dried hawthorn berries, water, honey **Preparation**: Simmer berries in water, strain, and sweeten with honey. **Storage**: Refrigerate for up to 2 weeks. **Usage**: Take 1 tablespoon twice daily. **Duration**: Consult a healthcare provider for long-term use. **Precautions**: Consult a doctor if you have heart conditions or are on medication.

Valerian Root Sleep Tincture

Ingredients: Dried valerian root, vodka **Preparation**: Soak valerian root in vodka for 4 weeks;

strain. **Storage**: Store in a dark bottle away from light; lasts up to 3 years. **Usage**: Take 1 ml 30 minutes before bedtime. **Duration**: Use for short-term sleep issues. **Precautions**: May cause drowsiness; avoid with sedatives.

Milk Thistle Seed Tea for Liver Detox

Ingredients: Milk thistle seeds, hot water **Preparation**: Crush seeds and steep in hot water for 20 minutes. **Storage**: Best consumed fresh; refrigerate for up to 24 hours. **Usage**: Drink 1 cup daily. **Duration**: Suitable for daily use. **Precautions**: Consult if you have a liver condition or are on medication.

Aloe Vera Gel for Skin Burns

Ingredients: Fresh aloe vera leaf **Preparation**: Slice leaf and extract the gel. **Storage**: Store gel in the refrigerator for up to 1 week. **Usage**: Apply to the burn as needed. **Duration**: Use until the burn heals.

Precautions: Test for allergic reaction on a small skin area.

Stinging Nettle Infusion for Allergy Relief

Ingredients: Dried stinging nettle leaves, hot water **Preparation**: Steep leaves in hot water for 10-15 minutes. **Storage**: Best consumed fresh; can refrigerate up to 24 hours. **Usage**: Drink 1-2 cups daily during allergy season. **Duration**: Suitable for daily use during allergy season. **Precautions**: May interact with blood pressure medication.

Catnip and Fennel Digestive Tea

Ingredients: Catnip leaves, fennel seeds, hot water **Preparation**: Steep leaves and seeds in hot water for 10 minutes. **Storage**: Best consumed fresh; refrigerate for up to 24 hours. **Usage**: Drink after meals as needed. **Duration**: Suitable for daily use. **Precautions**: Avoid if pregnant or nursing.

Yarrow Tincture for Fever Reduction

Ingredients: Yarrow flowers, vodka **Preparation**: Soak flowers in vodka for 4 weeks; strain. **Storage**: Store in a dark bottle away from light; lasts up to 3 years. **Usage**: Take 1 ml every 2-3 hours during fever. **Duration**: Use during fever episodes. **Precautions**: Not for prolonged use; avoid if pregnant.

Thyme Cough Syrup

Ingredients: Thyme leaves, honey, water **Preparation**: Simmer thyme in water, strain, and add honey. **Storage**: Refrigerate for up to 2 weeks. **Usage**: Take 1 teaspoon as needed for cough. **Duration**: Use as needed during cough. **Precautions**: Not for children under 1 year (due to honey).

Slippery Elm Lozenges for Sore Throat

Ingredients: Slippery elm bark powder, honey, water **Preparation**: Mix ingredients to form a dough, shape into lozenges, and dry. **Storage**: Store in a cool, dry place in an airtight container. **Usage**: Dissolve one lozenge in the mouth as needed. **Duration**: Use as needed for sore throat. **Precautions**: Ensure proper hydration while using.

Burdock Root Diuretic Tea

Ingredients: Burdock root, hot water **Preparation**: Steep sliced root in hot water for 15 minutes. **Storage**: Best consumed fresh; refrigerate for up to 24 hours. **Usage**: Drink 1 cup daily. **Duration**: Suitable for short-term use. **Precautions**: Avoid if dehydrated or on diuretics.

Sage Mouthwash for Oral Health

Ingredients: Sage leaves, water, optional: sea salt **Preparation**: Boil sage leaves in water, strain, and cool. Add sea salt if desired. **Storage**: Store in the refrigerator for up to 1 week. **Usage**: Rinse mouth twice daily. **Duration**: Suitable for daily use. **Precautions**: Avoid swallowing.

Passionflower Tea for Anxiety

Ingredients: Dried passionflower, hot water **Preparation**: Steep in hot water for 10 minutes. **Storage**: Best consumed fresh; refrigerate for up to 24 hours. **Usage**: Drink 1 cup in the evening or when anxious. **Duration**: Suitable for daily use. **Precautions**: May cause drowsiness; avoid with sedatives.

Rose Hip Immune-Boosting Tea

Ingredients: Dried rose hips, hot water **Preparation**: Steep in hot water for 15 minutes. **Storage**: Best consumed fresh; refrigerate for up to 24 hours. **Usage**: Drink 1-2 cups daily during cold seasons. **Duration**: Suitable for daily use during cold seasons. **Precautions**: High in vitamin C; monitor intake if on vitamin C supplements.

Ginkgo Biloba Tea for Memory Support

Ingredients: Dried ginkgo leaves, hot water **Preparation**: Steep in hot water for 10 minutes.

Storage: Best consumed fresh; refrigerate for up to 24 hours. **Usage**: Drink 1 cup daily. **Duration**: Consult a healthcare provider for long-term use. **Precautions**: May interact with blood thinners; avoid if on anticoagulant medication.

How to customize recipes for individual needs

Customizing herbal remedies to cater to individual needs is a cornerstone of effective herbal practice. While the recipes provided in this book are a great starting point, understanding how to tailor them to your unique requirements can significantly enhance their efficacy and safety. This sub-chapter guides you through the process of personalizing herbal recipes, ensuring that they align perfectly with your body's needs and your lifestyle.

Understanding Your Body and Health

1. **Listen to Your Body**: Pay attention to how your body responds to different herbs. Are there certain ingredients that seem more effective or cause discomfort? This awareness is crucial for customization.

2. **Identify Specific Needs**: Each individual has unique health needs based on factors like age, gender, lifestyle, and existing health conditions. Recognizing these needs helps tailor herbal remedies more effectively.

3. **Consult with a Professional**: If you have specific health concerns or are taking medication, consulting with a healthcare provider or a trained herbalist is vital. They can offer guidance on which herbs to use and which to avoid.

Adjusting Dosages

1. **Start Small**: When trying a new herb, begin with a lower dosage than recommended and gradually increase it. This approach helps gauge your body's reaction to the herb.

2. **Consider Age and Weight**: Dosages may need to be adjusted based on age and body weight. Children, seniors, and individuals with a smaller body mass typically require lower dosages.

3. **Monitor Effects**: Keep a journal to note the effects of different dosages. This record-keeping can help fine-tune the amount that works best for you.

Modifying Recipes

1. **Substitute Herbs**: If you're allergic to an herb or find it unpalatable, consider substitutes with similar properties. For example, if chamomile

doesn't suit you for stress relief, lemon balm might be an excellent alternative.

2. **Change Preparation Methods**: Depending on your preference and convenience, you might opt for a different preparation method. For instance, if you find teas cumbersome, tinctures or capsules might be better.

3. **Combine Remedies for Synergy**: Sometimes, combining two or more herbs can enhance their effectiveness. For example, combining ginger with turmeric can boost anti-inflammatory benefits. Always research or consult a professional to ensure the herbs you combine are safe together.

Lifestyle and Preference Considerations

1. **Flavor Adjustments**: Modify recipes to suit your taste preferences. Adding honey, lemon, or mint can improve the flavor of teas and infusions.

2. **Form Factor**: Choose a form that fits your lifestyle. If you're often on the go, capsules or tinctures might be more convenient than teas or decoctions.

3. **Allergies and Sensitivities**: Always consider allergies and sensitivities. If you're sensitive to a particular herb, finding an alternative or omitting it from a recipe is crucial.

Long-Term Adaptation

1. **Seasonal Adjustments**: Adapt your herbal regimen with the seasons. Some herbs are more suitable for certain times of the year, like elderberry during cold and flu season.

2. **Changing Health Needs**: As your health needs evolve, so should your herbal remedies. Regularly assess and adjust your herbal regimen to match your current health status.

3. **Continuous Learning**: Stay informed about herbal medicine. As research progresses, new

insights can help you further refine and improve your herbal practices.

By understanding and implementing these customization strategies, you can ensure that the herbal remedies you prepare are not only effective but also a joy to use. Personalization is about making herbal medicine work for you in the most harmonious way possible, enhancing your journey towards natural health and well-being.

Chapter
5

Chapter 5: Specialized Herbal Formulations

Advanced recipes for specific conditions (e.g., autoimmune disorders, chronic pain)

These recipes are designed to support individuals during and after intensive medical treatments. They emphasize gentle, supportive care, focusing on managing side effects, aiding recovery, and supporting overall well-being. In crafting these remedies, the focus has been on simplicity and effectiveness, ensuring they are safe, easy to prepare, and practical for everyday use. The detailed preparation steps, conservation details, precautions, and dosage information are aimed to empower the readers, allowing them to confidently incorporate these remedies into their health routines.

Chronic Inflammation: Rosehip and Boswellia Anti-Inflammatory Tea

Ingredients:

- 2 tbsp dried rosehip
- 1 tsp Boswellia powder
- Honey (optional)
- 1 liter of water

Preparation:

1. Boil water and add rosehips and Boswellia powder.
2. Simmer for 15 minutes.
3. Strain and add honey for taste if desired.

Conservation:

- Best consumed fresh; can be stored in the refrigerator for up to 2 days.

Precautions:

- Boswellia may interact with anti-inflammatory and cholesterol-lowering medications.

Dosage and Duration:

- Drink 1 cup daily for 6-8 weeks, then assess effectiveness.

Rheumatoid Arthritis: Willow Bark and Ginger Pain Relief Decoction

Ingredients:
- 1 tbsp dried willow bark
- 1 tsp grated fresh ginger
- 1 liter of water

Preparation:
1. Boil water with willow bark and ginger.
2. Simmer for 20 minutes.
3. Strain before drinking.

Conservation:
- Consume within 24 hours; store in a cool, dark place.

Precautions:
- Willow bark contains salicin; avoid if allergic to aspirin.
- Not suitable for children or pregnant women.

Dosage and Duration:

- Drink 1 cup once a day, preferably in the morning, for up to 6 weeks.

Psoriasis: Calendula and Chamomile Soothing Salve

Ingredients:

- 1/2 cup calendula petals
- 1/2 cup chamomile flowers
- 1 cup coconut oil
- 1/2 cup beeswax pellets

Preparation:

1. Gently heat coconut

oil in a double boiler and add calendula and chamomile. 2. Simmer on low heat for 1-2 hours, ensuring the oil doesn't overheat.

3. Strain the oil through a cheesecloth to remove the herbs.

4. Return the infused oil to the double boiler, add beeswax, and melt together.

5. Pour into small jars or tins and allow to cool and solidify.

Conservation:

- Store in a cool, dark place; the salve can last up to a year.

Precautions:

- Patch test on a small area of skin first to check for allergic reactions.

- Not recommended for use on open wounds or infected skin.

Dosage and Duration:

- Apply a small amount to affected areas once or twice daily. Continuous use for 2-3 weeks is recommended to see improvements.

Migraine Relief: Feverfew and Peppermint Tincture

Ingredients:

- 1 part dried feverfew leaves
- 1 part dried peppermint leaves
- Vodka or apple cider vinegar

Preparation:

1. Fill a jar 1/3 with a mixture of feverfew and peppermint.
2. Pour vodka or vinegar over the herbs, completely covering them.
3. Seal and store in a dark, cool place for 4 weeks, shaking daily.
4. Strain and bottle.

Conservation:

- Store the tincture in a cool, dark place; it can last for several years.

Precautions:

- Feverfew may interact with blood-thinning medications.
- Not recommended during pregnancy.

Dosage and Duration:

- Use 20-30 drops in water at the onset of migraine symptoms. Do not exceed 3 doses per day.

Chronic Fatigue: Ashwagandha and Licorice Root Adaptogen Blend

Ingredients:

- 2 tbsp ashwagandha root powder
- 1 tbsp licorice root powder
- 1 liter of water

Preparation:

1. Add ashwagandha and licorice root powder to boiling water.
2. Simmer for 15 minutes.
3. Strain and let it cool.

Conservation:

- Best consumed fresh, but can be refrigerated for up to 48 hours.

Precautions:

- Licorice root should not be used long-term or by individuals with hypertension.
- Consult a healthcare professional before using, especially if taking other medications.

Dosage and Duration:

- Drink 1 cup in the morning daily. Evaluate the benefits after 4-6 weeks of consistent use.

Post-Chemotherapy Nausea: Ginger and Lemon Balm Tea

Ingredients:

- 1 tsp fresh ginger, grated
- 1 tsp dried lemon balm
- 1 cup boiling water
- Honey (optional)

Preparation:

1. Steep ginger and lemon balm in boiling water for 10 minutes.
2. Strain and add honey if desired for taste.

Conservation:

- Consume fresh; if needed, store in the refrigerator for up to 12 hours.

Precautions:

- Consult your oncologist before using, as some herbs can interfere with chemotherapy.

Dosage and Duration:

- Sip slowly, 1 cup as needed for nausea, not exceeding 3 cups a day.

Cancer Recovery: Astragalus and Goji Berry Immune Booster

Ingredients:

- 2 tbsp dried astragalus root
- 1 tbsp dried goji berries
- 1 liter of water

Preparation:

1. Combine astragalus and goji berries with water and bring to a boil.
2. Simmer for 30 minutes.
3. Strain and serve warm.

Conservation:

- Best consumed fresh; can be stored in the refrigerator for up to 2 days.

Precautions:

- Always consult with your healthcare provider, especially when undergoing cancer treatment.

Dosage and Duration:

- Drink 1 cup daily for immune support during recovery.

Postoperative Recovery: Calendula and Lavender Healing Salve

Ingredients:

- ½ cup calendula petals
- ¼ cup lavender flowers
- 1 cup coconut oil
- ½ cup beeswax pellets

Preparation:

1. Infuse calendula and lavender in coconut oil over low heat for 2 hours.
2. Strain and add beeswax, melting all together.
3. Pour into containers and let cool to solidify.

Conservation:

- Store in a cool, dark place; can be used for up to 1 year.

Precautions:

- Use only on closed, healed wounds. Not for open or fresh post-surgical wounds.

Dosage and Duration:

- Apply gently to healed wounds 1-2 times daily as needed for comfort.

Chemotherapy Fatigue: Schisandra and Eleuthero Adaptogenic Tonic

Ingredients:

- 1 tbsp dried schisandra berries
- 1 tbsp dried eleuthero root
- 1 liter

of water

Preparation:

1. Combine schisandra berries and eleuthero root with water in a pot.

2. Bring to a boil, then reduce heat and simmer for 40 minutes.

3. Strain the mixture and allow it to cool.

Conservation:

- Best consumed fresh; refrigerate and use within 48 hours.

Precautions:

- Consult your oncologist before use, as some herbs may interact with chemotherapy medications.

- Eleuthero may increase blood pressure in some individuals.

Dosage and Duration:

- Drink 1 small cup (about 100 ml) in the morning. Observe for a week before continuing to ensure tolerability.

Post-Cancer Treatment: Dandelion Root Detox Tea

Ingredients:

- 2 tbsp dried dandelion root

- 1 liter of water
- Lemon or honey to taste (optional)

Preparation:

1. Simmer dandelion root in water for 15-20 minutes.
2. Strain and add lemon or honey if desired.

Conservation:

- Best consumed fresh; can be stored in the refrigerator for 24 hours.

Precautions:

- Dandelion can interact with certain medications, including diuretics and blood thinners.
- Consult with a healthcare provider before starting any new herbal regimen post-cancer treatment.

Dosage and Duration:

- Drink 1 cup daily, preferably in the morning, for up to 4 weeks, then take a break or reassess with a healthcare professional.

Recovery from Radiation Therapy: Aloe Vera and Chamomile Soothing Gel

Ingredients:

- 1 cup pure aloe vera gel
- 2 tbsp dried chamomile flowers
- 1 cup distilled water

Preparation:

1. Steep chamomile flowers in boiling water for 15 minutes.
2. Strain and mix the chamomile infusion with the aloe vera gel.
3. Store in a clean container.

Conservation:

- Keep refrigerated and use within one week for maximum freshness.

Precautions:

- Perform a patch test on a small skin area first to check for any allergic reaction.
- Apply only on skin areas affected by radiation therapy and not on open wounds.

Dosage and Duration:

- Gently apply to affected skin areas 2-3 times daily, especially after bathing or as needed for comfort.

Blending herbs for synergistic effects

This sub-chapter delves into the principles and practices of herbal blending, providing guidance on how to combine different herbs to enhance their therapeutic effects and create remedies that are greater than the sum of their parts.

Synergy occurs when the interaction of herbs results in a therapeutic effect that is more potent than what each herb could achieve individually. This synergy can amplify the desired effects, mitigate potential side effects, and even target multiple symptoms or causes of a condition simultaneously. Understanding the properties, actions, and energetics of each herb is crucial for creating effective blends.

Principles of Herbal Blending

1. **Complementary Actions**: Select herbs that complement each other's actions. For instance, combining a soothing herb like chamomile with a digestive aid like ginger can create a blend that both calms and supports digestion.

2. **Balancing Energetics**: Herbs have energetic qualities such as warming, cooling, drying, or moistening. A well-crafted blend balances these energetics to suit the individual's constitution and the nature of their condition. For example, a blend for inflammation might include both cooling herbs to reduce heat and warming herbs to stimulate circulation.

3. **Layering Flavors**: The taste of an herbal blend can influence its therapeutic effect. Bitter herbs stimulate digestion, sweet herbs can be nourishing, and pungent herbs may promote circulation. Balancing these flavors makes the

remedy more palatable and can enhance its efficacy.

4. **Targeting Multiple Systems**: Many conditions affect multiple body systems. A blend might include an herb that targets the primary concern and others that support secondary systems. In a blend for stress, you might include an adaptogen for overall stress resistance and a nervine to specifically soothe the nervous system.

Steps for Crafting Synergistic Blends

1. **Identify the Primary Concern**: Define the main health issue you are addressing. Choose one or two primary herbs that directly target this concern.

2. **Select Supportive Herbs**: Add herbs that support the primary action or target related symptoms or systems. These should complement and enhance the primary herbs.

3. **Consider the Dosage and Form**: Decide on the form of your remedy (tea, tincture, capsule) and adjust the proportions of each herb accordingly. Some herbs may be stronger or more effective in certain forms.

4. **Test and Adjust**: Start with small batches and adjust the ratios based on effectiveness and taste. Personal experience and feedback are invaluable in fine-tuning a blend.

5. **Record Your Recipes**: Keep detailed notes on the herbs, proportions, and effects of your blends. This documentation is essential for replicating successful blends and understanding the nuances of herbal synergies.

Example Blends for Common Conditions

- **Sleep Support Blend**: Lavender (calming), Chamomile (relaxant), Valerian root (sedative), and Lemon balm (mood support). This blend addresses multiple facets of sleep issues, from anxiety to physical relaxation.

- **Digestive Aid Blend**: Peppermint (antispasmodic), Fennel seeds (carminative), Ginger (digestive stimulant), and Slippery elm (soothing mucilage). This combination can help alleviate various digestive discomforts, including gas, bloating, and irritation.

- **Immune Boosting Blend**: Echinacea (immune stimulant), Elderberry (antiviral), Astragalus (deep immune support), and Ginger (warming and stimulating). This blend covers immediate immune response and longer-term immune health.

chapter

6

Chapter 6: Dosage, Safety, and Efficacy

Determining effective dosages for different herbs

It's akin to finding the perfect balance in a delicate dance – too little, and the dance lacks grace; too much, and it becomes overbearing. This balance is especially crucial considering our target audience – well-educated, middle-aged women who are attuned to the subtleties of integrated natural medicine and seek practical, easy-to-understand information that can be seamlessly incorporated into their busy lives.

The process of establishing the right dosage of an herb is both an art and a science. It's a science because it involves understanding the pharmacological aspects of herbs, their active constituents, and how they interact with the human body. It's an art because each individual's response to herbs can vary based on factors like age, weight, health status, and even genetic makeup.

When determining dosages, one must consider the herb's potency, the condition being treated, the individual's characteristics, and the form in which the herb will be used. For instance, a tincture might require a different dosage than a tea or a capsule.

Factors Influencing Dosage

Potency of the Herb: Some herbs, like valerian or kava, are potent and require smaller doses. Others, like chamomile or lavender, can be used in relatively larger amounts. Understanding the strength of each herb is crucial.

Individual's Health Status: The presence of chronic conditions, allergies, or sensitivities can affect how an individual responds to an herb. For example, someone with a sensitive stomach might require a lower dose of a potent digestive herb like cayenne.

Age and Weight Considerations: Generally, dosages are calculated based on an average adult of a certain weight range. Adjustments are made for children, the elderly, and individuals who are significantly under or overweight.

Form of the Herb: The form in which an herb is administered – tea, tincture, capsule, extract – has a significant impact on its dosage. Concentrated forms like extracts and tinctures are used in smaller quantities than teas or infusions.

Establishing Dosages: A Step-by-Step Approach

Begin with Research: Investigate the standard recommended dosages for the herb in question. Resources like herbal textbooks, peer-reviewed journals, and reputable online databases can provide a solid starting point.

Consider the Application: Are you creating a remedy for acute symptoms, like a headache or indigestion, or for chronic conditions like arthritis or insomnia? Acute conditions may require higher dosages for a short duration, whereas chronic conditions often call for lower, more consistent dosages over time.

Adjust for Individual Needs: Take into account the individual's unique characteristics. For instance, a smaller, more sensitive person might start at the lower end of the dosage range, while someone larger and less sensitive may require a higher dose.

Account for Herb Forms: If using tinctures, start with the number of drops recommended by reliable sources, usually ranging from 20 to 40 drops. For teas, a standard dose might be one teaspoon of dried herb per cup of boiling water, steeped for 10 to 15 minutes. Capsules and tablets should follow the manufacturer's or a trusted herbalist's recommendation.

Monitor and Adjust: Initial dosages should be seen as a starting point. Close monitoring of the effects and any side effects is crucial. Adjust the dosage as needed based on the individual's response.

Consultation with Healthcare Professionals: Especially in cases of chronic conditions or when other medications are involved, consulting with a healthcare professional is vital. They can provide guidance on potential herb-drug interactions and other safety considerations.

Practical Examples in Dosage Determination

Lavender for Stress Relief: Lavender is relatively gentle and can be used in various forms. A standard dose for tea might be 1-2 teaspoons of dried flowers per cup of hot water. For a tincture, 30-40 drops in water or juice up to three times a day can be calming.

Turmeric for Inflammation: The active compound in turmeric, curcumin, is potent. Standard dosages might range from 400 to 600 mg of powdered root in capsules three times a day. As a tea, one might use 1-2 grams of the dried, powdered root steeped in boiling water.

Echinacea for Immune Support: For echinacea, dosages can vary based on the form and species of the herb. For a tincture of Echinacea purpurea, a general dose might be 2-4 ml up to three times a day at the onset of cold or flu symptoms.

Safety guidelines and contraindications

In the practice of herbal medicine, safety is paramount. While herbs offer a natural path to healing and wellness, they are not without risks. Understanding safety guidelines and being aware of contraindications is essential for anyone using herbal remedies. This chapter is dedicated to providing comprehensive safety information to ensure that your journey with herbal medicine is both effective and secure.

The allure of herbal medicine lies in its accessibility and perceived gentleness, but this should not lead to complacency regarding its use. Herbs, like any medicinal substances, have the potential to cause adverse effects if used improperly. As a practitioner or user of herbal medicine, you bear the responsibility of understanding these risks and using herbs wisely.

Understanding Herb-Drug Interactions

One of the critical aspects of herbal safety is understanding potential interactions between herbal remedies and pharmaceutical drugs. Herbs can augment, diminish, or otherwise alter the effects of prescription medications. For instance, St. John's Wort, known for its antidepressant properties, can reduce the effectiveness of certain prescription drugs, including birth control pills and some types of cancer medications.

It is crucial to consult with a healthcare professional, ideally someone knowledgeable in both conventional and herbal medicine, before combining herbs with prescription medications. This consultation is not just a formality; it is a vital step in ensuring your health and safety.

Recognizing Allergic Reactions and Sensitivities

Just as some individuals are allergic to certain foods or environmental elements, the same can be true for herbs. An allergic reaction to an herb can range from mild – such as a skin rash or hives – to severe, like anaphylaxis. Knowing your body's reactions and being alert to new symptoms when trying a new herb is important.

When starting with any new herbal remedy, it is advisable to begin with a small dose and monitor for any adverse reactions. This cautious approach is particularly important for individuals known to have multiple allergies or sensitivities.

Dosage Considerations

The principle of "start low and go slow" is wise to follow in herbal medicine. The correct dosage of an herbal remedy can vary significantly depending on factors like age, weight, health condition, and the specific herb being used. Overdosing on certain herbs can lead to negative side effects. For example, excessive use of licorice root can lead to hypertension and low potassium levels.

It is essential to adhere to recommended dosages provided by reliable sources and not to exceed them without professional guidance. In herbal medicine, more is not necessarily better; often, smaller, consistent doses are more effective and safer.

Special Populations: Pregnancy, Breastfeeding, and Children

Certain herbs should be avoided during pregnancy and breastfeeding due to potential risks to the baby. For instance, herbs like pennyroyal or goldenseal are considered unsafe during pregnancy. Similarly, while using herbal remedies for children, one must be extremely cautious as their bodies process substances differently than adults.

Consultation with a healthcare provider is non-negotiable for these sensitive groups. When it comes to the health of a child or an unborn baby, professional guidance is paramount in avoiding potential risks.

Understanding the Long-Term Use of Herbs

While some herbs can be safely used over long periods, others are meant for short-term use only. For example, cascara sagrada, a natural laxative, should not be used for extended periods as it can lead to dependency and loss of bowel function.

Knowing the long-term effects of any herbal remedy is crucial. Continuous use of certain herbs can lead to an imbalance in the body's natural systems. It's important to research and understand the ideal duration of use for any herbal remedy and to take breaks when necessary.

Navigating the World of Herbal Supplements

The market is flooded with herbal supplements, and not all are created equal. The quality, potency, and purity of herbal supplements can vary widely between brands. Some may contain additives or contaminants, or they may not contain the advertised herb at all.

It is essential to choose high-quality, reputable brands for herbal supplements. Look for products that have been independently tested and verified for quality. Additionally, understanding the labeling and potency of these supplements is crucial for safe use.

Chapter

7

Chapter 7: Herbal Remedies for Mental and Emotional Well-being

Herbs for stress relief, anxiety, and sleep disorders

These conditions, so prevalent in our fast-paced modern world, often intertwine, impacting one's overall well-being. This section provides a deep dive into the herbal remedies specifically tailored to address these concerns, offering a natural path to tranquility and restorative sleep. We'll explore various herbs, their preparations, dosages, and necessary precautions, ensuring a comprehensive understanding for effective use.

Lavender for General Anxiety

Renowned for its calming scent, lavender is a go-to herb for anxiety relief. A simple preparation is a lavender tea or infusion, using 1-2 teaspoons of dried lavender per cup of boiling water. Steep for 10 minutes and enjoy up to twice daily. Lavender is generally safe, but excessive use can lead to drowsiness.

Chamomile for Stress-Induced Upset Stomach

Chamomile is not only soothing for the mind but also for the digestive system. Prepare a chamomile tea by steeping 2-3 teaspoons of dried flowers in hot water for 5 minutes. Drink 1-2 cups in the evening or when experiencing stress-related digestive discomfort. Avoid chamomile if you are allergic to plants in the daisy family.

Ashwagandha for Chronic Stress

Ashwagandha, an adaptogen, helps the body resist stressors. The typical dose is about 300-500 mg of root extract, taken once or twice daily. It's best to start with a lower dose to assess tolerance. Pregnant women should avoid ashwagandha.

Lemon Balm for Nervous Tension

Lemon balm can alleviate nervous tension and improve mood. To prepare, steep 2 teaspoons of dried lemon balm in hot water for 10 minutes. It's safe for daily use, but high doses may cause dizziness in some individuals.

Passionflower for Anxiety and Sleep Troubles

Passionflower can be particularly effective for those whose anxiety interferes with sleep. Use about 1 teaspoon of dried herb per cup of boiling water, steeping for 10 minutes. Limit intake to once in the evening as it can cause drowsiness.

Valerian Root for Anxiety-Related Insomnia

Valerian root is potent for sleep disturbances related to anxiety. Take 300-600 mg of valerian root extract about an hour before bedtime. Note that it might take two weeks to experience full benefits. Avoid operating heavy machinery after consumption due to its sedative effects.

Managing Sleep Disorders: Herbal Solutions for Restful Nights

Hops for Sleeplessness

Hops, often associated with beer, are excellent for inducing sleep. A simple hops pillow or a tea made from 1-2 teaspoons of dried hops steeped for 10 minutes before bedtime can be effective. Hops should be used cautiously as they can exacerbate depressive symptoms in some individuals.

Skullcap for Restlessness

Skullcap is a nerve tonic that can alleviate restlessness and insomnia. Prepare a tea with 1-2 teaspoons of dried skullcap, steeping for 10 minutes. Drink it in the evening to promote relaxation and sleep.

California Poppy for Sleep Disturbance

California poppy acts as a mild sedative. Prepare a tea using 1-2 teaspoons of the herb per cup of hot water. It's particularly effective when combined with other sedative herbs like valerian.

Magnolia Bark for REM Sleep

Magnolia bark can enhance the quality of REM sleep. Use around 200-400 mg of magnolia extract before bedtime. Pregnant or breastfeeding women should avoid magnolia bark.

St. John's Wort for Sleep Disruption Due to Depression

St. John's Wort is known for its antidepressant properties and can aid sleep. The standard dose is 300 mg of extract three times daily. It's important to note that St. John's Wort can interact with various medications, including antidepressants.

Catnip for Gentle Sleep Aid

Catnip, not just for cats, can be a gentle sleep aid. Brew a tea with 1-2 teaspoons of dried catnip leaves steeped in hot water for 10 minutes. It's safe for nightly use and is particularly suitable for children.

Creating a holistic mental health regimen

Mental health is a complex interplay of physical, emotional, environmental, and nutritional factors. Understanding this interconnectivity and addressing all aspects can lead to a more balanced, healthier state of mind. This chapter explores how to create a comprehensive mental health regimen that encompasses herbs, diet, sleep, hydration, air quality, and emotional management.

The Interconnected Nature of Mental Well-being

Our mental health does not exist in a vacuum. It is deeply influenced by our physical health, the food we eat, the air we breathe, our sleep patterns, our hydration levels, and, crucially, how we manage our emotions. A holistic approach recognizes these connections and seeks to harmonize them.

Nourishment for the Mind

What we eat profoundly impacts our mental health. Foods rich in omega-3 fatty acids, such as salmon and flaxseeds, are known for their brain-boosting properties. Complex carbohydrates, found in whole grains, provide a steady release of glucose to the brain, enhancing cognitive function and mood stability. Leafy greens, nuts, and seeds are rich in magnesium, a mineral that plays a crucial role in regulating neurotransmitters, which in turn affect mood and stress levels.

Incorporating these foods into your daily diet can support mental well-being. Remember, the aim is not to overhaul your diet overnight but to make gradual, sustainable changes that can be maintained in the long term.

The Healing Power of Sleep

Sleep is a critical component of mental health. It's during sleep that our brains process the day's events, consolidate memories, and restore themselves. Lack of quality sleep can lead to irritability, difficulty concentrating, and exacerbate mental health issues.

Creating a sleep-conducive environment is key. This includes maintaining a regular sleep schedule, ensuring your bedroom is dark, quiet, and cool, and avoiding screens at least an hour before bed. Herbs like valerian root and lavender can be used in teas or as essential oils to promote relaxation and improve sleep quality.

Hydration: A Simple Yet Powerful Tool

Often overlooked, hydration is vital for mental health. Even mild dehydration can impair cognitive function, mood, and energy levels. The brain is approximately 75% water, and maintaining this hydration is essential for its optimal function.

Drinking water throughout the day, infused with herbs like lemon balm or mint, can be a refreshing way to stay hydrated and boost your mental energy.

Breathing in Good Health

The air we breathe can significantly impact our mental clarity and stress levels. Poor air quality, both indoors and outdoors, can contribute to cognitive decline and mental fatigue. Ensuring good ventilation in your living spaces, using air purifiers, and surrounding yourself with air-purifying plants like spider plants or peace lilies can enhance the air quality. Additionally, practices like deep breathing or using a neti pot can help clear your airways and improve oxygen flow to the brain, enhancing mental clarity.

Managing Emotions through Mindfulness

Emotional management is perhaps the most personalized aspect of mental health. Techniques like mindfulness, meditation, and journaling can be profoundly effective in understanding and regulating emotions. Mindfulness helps in grounding your thoughts in the present, reducing anxiety and stress. Meditation, even for a few minutes a day, can improve focus and bring a sense of calm. Journaling provides an outlet for expressing thoughts and emotions, offering clarity and perspective.

Herbs like ashwagandha and rhodiola can be incorporated to help manage stress and improve resilience to emotional stressors. However, the key is to find practices that resonate with you personally and integrate them into your daily routine.

Putting It All Together

Creating a holistic mental health regimen is not about perfection; it's about balance and integration. Start by incorporating one or two changes, like adjusting your diet or introducing a sleep ritual, and gradually build from there. Remember, the goal is to create a sustainable lifestyle that supports your mental and emotional well-being.

In summary, mental health is multifaceted, and its care should be equally comprehensive. By combining nutritional support, sleep hygiene, proper hydration, quality air, and emotional management techniques, along with the judicious use of herbs, you can create a robust foundation for mental and emotional well-being. This holistic approach empowers you to take control of your mental health, leading to a more balanced, fulfilling life.

Chapter

8

Chapter 8: The Herbal Kitchen

Incorporating medicinal herbs into daily cooking

Integrating medicinal herbs into daily cooking is not just about enhancing flavor. It's about transforming everyday meals into opportunities for health and wellness. This sub-chapter is dedicated to guiding you through the versatile and enjoyable ways of incorporating medicinal herbs into your regular cooking routine. Here, we'll explore methods to infuse these potent plants into your daily diet, making each meal a step towards better health.

Embracing Herbs in Everyday Cuisine

The beauty of cooking with medicinal herbs lies in their versatility. Whether it's a busy weekday dinner or a leisurely weekend brunch, herbs can be seamlessly added to a wide array of dishes, imparting both flavor and therapeutic benefits. Let's explore how to make herbs a staple in your kitchen.

Breakfast: A Herbal Start to Your Day

Starting your day with a herb-infused breakfast can set a positive tone for your health. Consider adding herbs to your morning smoothies, oatmeal, or eggs. For instance, a smoothie with spinach, parsley, and mint offers a refreshing and detoxifying start. Sprinkling cinnamon on your oatmeal can help regulate blood sugar levels, while adding basil to your scrambled eggs can provide an anti-inflammatory boost.

Lunch: Herbs in Salads, Soups, and Sandwiches

Lunch is a perfect time to incorporate a variety of fresh herbs. Adding herbs like dill, cilantro, or chives to salads not only enhances flavor but also boosts digestive health. Soups and stews can be enriched with herbs such as rosemary, thyme, and oregano, which offer antimicrobial and immune-boosting properties. For sandwiches, consider spreads like basil pesto or a thyme and garlic aioli, which pack both flavor and health benefits.

Dinner: Robust Flavors and Healing Properties

Dinner is an ideal time to experiment with more robust herbal flavors. Incorporating herbs into marinades and sauces can transform a simple meal. For instance, marinating chicken or fish with a blend of sage, lemon, and garlic not only imparts a wonderful flavor but also supports digestion and immunity. Adding herbs like turmeric and ginger to your stir-fries can offer anti-inflammatory benefits. Even a simple garnish of parsley can provide a burst of vitamins and aid in detoxification.

Snacks and Desserts: A Herbal Twist

Snacks and desserts are often overlooked as opportunities to include medicinal herbs. Adding fresh mint or basil to fruit salads can aid digestion and add an interesting flavor profile. Creating desserts with lavender or chamomile can provide a calming effect, perfect for winding down in the evening.

Beverages: Sipping on Health

Herbs can play a significant role in your hydration habits. Infusing water with herbs like mint, cucumber, and lemon not only makes for a refreshing drink but also aids in digestion and detoxification. Herbal teas, such as chamomile, peppermint, or ginger tea, are excellent for soothing the digestive system and calming the mind.

The Art of Seasoning: Finding the Right Balance

Seasoning with herbs is an art that enhances the health benefits and flavors of your food. It's important to find the right balance where the herbs complement rather than overpower the dish. Fresh herbs usually have a milder flavor than dried ones and are best added towards the end of the cooking process to preserve their flavor and health properties.

Growing Your Herbal Pantry

Having a variety of fresh herbs at your disposal can inspire regular use in your cooking. Consider growing a small herb garden in your kitchen or balcony. Herbs like basil, mint, cilantro, and parsley are easy to grow and maintain. Not only do they provide fresh, organic herbs for your cooking, but they also bring a bit of nature into your home.

Recipes for infusions, smoothies and culinary delights

Creating herbal culinary delights is an art that blends taste, health, and creativity. This sub-chapter will explore a variety of unique and wholesome recipes, including herbal teas, infusions, smoothies, salads, and desserts. Each recipe is designed to offer both health benefits and culinary enjoyment, using a mix of herbs, fruits, and vegetables to create flavors that are both delightful and beneficial. Each of these recipes is designed to be both healthful and flavorful, integrating the healing properties of herbs into everyday meals and beverages. They offer a delightful way to incorporate natural remedies into a balanced lifestyle, providing benefits that extend beyond just taste.

Peppermint and Pineapple Smoothie

Ingredients:

1 cup fresh pineapple, diced

½ cup peppermint leaves

1 banana

1 cup almond milk

Procedure: Blend all ingredients until smooth.

Benefits: Energizing and aids digestion.

Lavender and Lemon Infusion

Ingredients:

1 tsp dried lavender flowers

Juice of 1 lemon

1 tsp honey

Procedure: Steep lavender in hot water for 5 minutes. Strain, add lemon juice and honey.

Benefits: Calming and soothing for the nerves.

Thyme and Citrus Salad

Ingredients:

2 cups mixed greens

1 orange, segmented

1 grapefruit, segmented

2 tbsp fresh thyme, chopped

Olive oil and balsamic vinegar for dressing

Procedure: Combine all ingredients and toss with dressing.

Benefits: Boosts immunity and provides vitamin C.

Basil and Berry Herbal Mousse

Ingredients:

1 cup fresh basil leaves

2 cups mixed berries

1 cup Greek yogurt

2 tbsp honey

Procedure: Blend basil with berries, yogurt, and honey until smooth. Chill before serving.

Benefits: Rich in antioxidants and aids digestion.

Sage and Apple Infused Water

Ingredients:

1 apple, thinly sliced

5 sage leaves

1 liter of water

Procedure: Combine all ingredients in a pitcher and refrigerate for at least 2 hours.

Benefits: Hydrating and improves cognitive function.

Rosemary and Peach Iced Tea

Ingredients:

4 peach tea bags

1 sprig of rosemary

Honey to taste

Procedure: Steep tea bags and rosemary in boiling water, then chill. Add honey to taste.

Benefits: Refreshing and aids memory.

Mint and Cucumber Salad

Ingredients:

2 cucumbers, sliced

½ cup mint leaves, chopped

Lemon juice and olive oil for dressing

Procedure: Toss cucumbers and mint with lemon juice and olive oil.

Benefits: Cooling and hydrating.

Ginger and Turmeric Smoothie

Ingredients:

1 inch fresh ginger, grated

1 tsp turmeric powder

1 banana

1 cup coconut milk

Procedure: Blend all ingredients until smooth.

Benefits: Anti-inflammatory and boosts immunity.

Dandelion Green and Walnut Salad

Ingredients:

2 cups dandelion greens, chopped

½ cup walnuts, toasted

¼ cup dried cranberries

Olive oil and apple cider vinegar for dressing

Procedure: Combine ingredients and dress lightly.

Benefits: Detoxifying and rich in omega-3.

Chamomile and Honey Panna Cotta

Ingredients:

2 cups cream

1 tbsp dried chamomile flowers

¼ cup honey

1 tsp gelatin

Procedure: Infuse chamomile in warm cream, strain, and add honey and gelatin. Set in molds.

Benefits: Soothing and aids sleep.

Lemon Balm and Blueberry Infusion

Ingredients:

1 cup blueberries

½ cup lemon balm leaves

1 liter of water

Procedure: Muddle blueberries and lemon balm in water, refrigerate overnight.

Benefits: Refreshing and stress-reducing.

Fennel and Orange Salad

Ingredients:

1 fennel bulb, thinly sliced

2 oranges, segmented

Arugula

Olive oil and lemon juice for dressing

Procedure: Combine fennel, oranges, and arugula. Dress lightly.

Benefits: Digestive aid and rich in vitamin C.

Rose Petal and Strawberry Smoothie

Ingredients:

1 cup strawberries

2 tbsp dried rose petals

1 cup almond milk

1 tbsp honey

Procedure: Blend all ingredients until smooth.

Benefits: Heart-healthy and mood-enhancing.

Cilantro and Lime Infused Water

Ingredients:

1 bunch cilantro

Juice of 2 limes

1 liter of water

Procedure: Combine cilantro and lime juice in water, refrigerate for 2 hours.

Benefits: Detoxifying and aids digestion.

Hibiscus and Raspberry Iced Tea

Ingredients:

¼ cup dried hibiscus flowers

1 cup raspberries

Honey to taste

Procedure: Steep hibiscus and raspberries in boiling water, then chill. Add honey.

Benefits: High in antioxidants and refreshing.

Parsley and Quinoa Tabbouleh

Ingredients:

1 cup quinoa, cooked

1 cup parsley, finely chopped

½ cup mint, chopped

Tomatoes, cucumbers, lemon juice, and olive oil

Procedure: Combine all ingredients. Add lemon juice and olive oil to taste.

Benefits: Rich in vitamins and minerals, aids detoxification.

Lavender and Honey Glazed Carrots

Ingredients:

6 carrots, sliced

2 tbsp honey

1 tsp dried lavender

Butter

Procedure: Sauté carrots in butter, honey, and lavender until tender.

Benefits: Soothing and good for digestion.

Nettle and Potato Soup

Ingredients:

2 cups nettle leaves, blanched

4 potatoes, cubed

Onion, garlic, vegetable broth

Procedure: Sauté onion and garlic, add potatoes and broth. Add nettles, simmer until potatoes are soft.

Benefits: Rich in iron and supports joint health.

Elderflower and Lemon Sorbet

Ingredients:

½ cup elderflower syrup

Juice of 2 lemons

2 cups water

Sugar to taste

Procedure: Combine ingredients, freeze, and stir occasionally until set.

Benefits: Immune-boosting and refreshing.

Thyme and Apple Compote

Ingredients:

4 apples, peeled and diced

2 tbsp thyme leaves

Sugar and water as needed

Procedure: Simmer apples, thyme, sugar, and water until apples are soft.

Benefits: Aids digestion and is rich in antioxidants.

chapter
9

Chapter 9: Herbal Care for Women, Men, and Children

Tailoring herbal remedies for different genders and ages

The nuances in physiological and psychological makeup across various life stages and between genders significantly influence how individuals respond to herbal treatments. This chapter delves into these distinctions, offering insights into crafting herbal remedies that honor and cater to these differences.

Men's Health: Beyond the Stereotypes

The narrative of men's health often revolves around vigor and vitality, overlooking the subtleties of emotional and mental well-being. Saw Palmetto is renowned for its support in prostate health, a significant concern for many men as they age. But men's herbal health goes beyond the physical. Adaptogens like Rhodiola can be particularly beneficial for men, offering support for stress management and mental clarity – two aspects that are often overlooked in the male health paradigm.

Children: The Delicate Art of Pediatric Herbalism

When it comes to children, gentleness is key. Their bodies are still developing, and their physiological responses to herbs can be quite different from adults. For common childhood ailments like colds and stomach upsets, relying on mild herbs like Elderflower and Chamomile can be both safe and effective. Dosage, of course, is a critical consideration – it should be carefully adjusted according to age and weight.

The teenage years bring a set of challenges unique to this developmental stage. Herbs that support concentration and reduce stress, such as Lemon

Balm, can be particularly beneficial for teenagers navigating the pressures of academic life and social changes.

Aging Gracefully: Herbal Support in Elder Years

As we age, our bodies require different types of support. Herbs can play a vital role in promoting vitality, cognitive function, and joint health. Ginkgo Biloba, for instance, is celebrated for its ability to enhance cognitive function, while Turmeric is a favorite for its anti-inflammatory properties, particularly beneficial for joint health.

However, it's not just about physical health. The elder years can also bring feelings of isolation or sadness. Herbs that support emotional well-being, such as St. John's Wort, can be invaluable during this life stage, offering a gentle way to uplift the spirit.

Women's Herbal Health: A Journey Through Life Stages

The journey of women's health is inherently linked to the natural rhythms of life – from the onset of menstruation to the transition of menopause. Each stage brings its unique challenges and opportunities for growth, and herbal medicine provides a gentle, yet powerful, means to navigate these transitions.

Menstrual Health: Balancing the Cycle

The menstrual cycle is a barometer of overall health for many women. During the reproductive years, managing menstrual health is not just about alleviating symptoms but also about maintaining a balance. Herbs like Chaste Tree (Vitex agnus-castus) play a crucial role in this. Vitex, known for its hormone-balancing properties, can help regulate irregular cycles and ease premenstrual symptoms such as mood swings and bloating. Red Raspberry

Leaf, a uterine tonic, is another ally, supporting uterine health and easing menstrual cramps. These herbs, however, are not just remedies; they are tools that empower women to understand and harmonize with their bodies' natural rhythms.

Pregnancy: A Time of Gentle Nurturance

Pregnancy is a time of profound transformation, requiring a delicate balance of nurturing the mother and the developing child. Gentle herbs like Ginger are invaluable for managing morning sickness, while Red Raspberry Leaf again plays a role in supporting uterine health, potentially aiding in smoother labor. It's important to note, however, that not all herbs are safe during pregnancy. The use of herbal medicine during this time should be approached with care, consulting healthcare professionals to ensure safety for both mother and baby.

Postpartum Care: Nourishing the New Mother

The postpartum period is often a time of immense change and adjustment. Herbs can be a source of comfort and healing during this time. Motherwort is known for its ability to ease postpartum blues and support heart health, while Nettle provides a rich source of nutrients to help replenish a mother's body. The focus here is not just on physical recovery, but also on emotional well-being, acknowledging the profound journey of becoming a mother.

Menopause: Embracing Change with Grace

Menopause marks a significant transition in a woman's life, often accompanied by a range of physical and emotional changes. Black Cohosh and Dong Quai are renowned for their ability to alleviate menopausal symptoms like hot flashes and mood swings. These herbs, however, do more than just relieve symptoms; they support a woman in embracing this new phase of life. Menopause is not just an end to fertility, but a beginning of a new era of wisdom and freedom.

Holistic Support for All Stages

In every stage of a woman's life, herbs offer more than just physical remedies – they provide a way to connect with the wisdom of nature and one's own body. This holistic approach acknowledges the physical, emotional, and spiritual dimensions of health, offering support that is nurturing, empowering, and deeply healing.

Considerations for Pregnancy, Menstrual Health, and Menopause

Pregnancy is a time when the body undergoes significant changes, and the need for safe, natural support is paramount. Herbs like Raspberry Leaf and Nettle not only offer nutritional support but also prepare the body for childbirth. However, the key is to use these herbs under guidance, understanding which herbs are safe and in what quantities.

The approach to **menstrual health** in herbal medicine goes beyond just managing symptoms. It's about understanding the underlying imbalances and addressing them holistically. For instance, herbs like Evening Primrose Oil can help in regulating hormonal imbalances, while herbs like Cramp Bark offer relief from menstrual cramps, addressing the immediate discomfort.

Menopause, often fraught with mixed emotions and physical discomfort, can be a time of revitalization with the right herbal support. Herbs like Sage can help in reducing night sweats, while Red Clover may offer benefits for bone health, which becomes a concern during this stage. This period is also an opportunity to focus on heart health and emotional well-being, using herbs like Hawthorn and Lemon Balm.

Chapter
10

Chapter 10: Building an Herbal Medicine Cabinet

This chapter is dedicated to guiding you through the process of creating a space in your home where nature's remedies meet your family's health needs. Whether you're a novice to herbalism or a seasoned practitioner, having a well-stocked, thoughtfully curated herbal medicine cabinet is indispensable.

The art of assembling an herbal medicine cabinet goes beyond mere collection. It's about understanding the herbs that resonate with your and your family's specific health needs and lifestyles. This chapter will serve as your roadmap, helping you navigate through the vast world of herbal remedies, selecting those that will form the cornerstone of your natural healthcare.

We'll explore the essentials for a beginner's herbal medicine kit, providing recommendations for versatile, safe, and effective herbs that address a wide range of common ailments. From soothing digestive issues to calming a restless mind, from boosting immunity to relieving pain, these foundational herbs are your allies in everyday health.

As we delve deeper, you'll learn about the art of preservation and storage, ensuring that the potency and efficacy of your herbs are maintained. Proper storage is crucial in herbal medicine, as it safeguards the integrity and therapeutic value of the herbs. We'll cover various methods, from drying and tincturing to oil infusions and proper container selection, equipping you with the knowledge to keep your herbs vibrant and effective.

Moreover, this chapter isn't just about what goes into your cabinet, but also how you integrate this knowledge into your daily life.

Essentials for a home herbal medicine kit

In the creation of a home herbal medicine kit, while the herbs themselves are of paramount importance, the tools and storage methods you choose are equally crucial in determining the efficacy and longevity of your remedies. This comprehensive guide takes you through the essential tools for both the preparation and storage of your herbal remedies, ensuring that they maintain their potency and purity.

For Harvesting:

- **Pruning Shears**: Essential for a clean and precise cut, these shears minimize damage to plants, promoting healthy regrowth.
- **Gloves**: Protecting your hands is crucial, especially when handling herbs that may have thorns or cause skin irritation.
- **Baskets or Cloth Bags**: Preferable to plastic, these allow air circulation, preventing wilting or mold.
- **Field Guide**: Invaluable for correctly identifying herbs and understanding their natural habitats.

For Processing Herbs:

- **Mortar and Pestle**: A timeless tool, indispensable for grinding and blending herbs to unlock their full spectrum of flavors and medicinal properties.

- **Herb Drying Racks**: Vital for properly drying herbs, these racks ensure even air circulation, crucial for preservation.

- **Saucepan and Double Boiler**: Essential for making decoctions, teas, and infused oils, they allow for controlled heating, preserving the beneficial compounds of the herbs.

- **Strainers and Cheesecloth**: Necessary for filtering tinctures or teas, ensuring clarity and purity in your preparations.

Tools for Preparation and Storage

- **Glass Jars and Bottles**: Indispensable for storing tinctures, teas, and infused oils. Amber or cobalt glass bottles offer additional protection from light.

- **Measuring Cups and Spoons**: Ensure accuracy in herbal preparation, maintaining the balance and effectiveness of your remedies.

- **Funnel**: Often overlooked, a funnel is invaluable for transferring liquids like tinctures and oils into storage bottles, ensuring a mess-free process.

- **Glass Jars for Infusion**: Key for infusing oils or creating tinctures, these jars should be of high quality to withstand prolonged use.

Long-term storage and preservation of herbs

The art of preserving herbs is as ancient as herbal medicine itself. It is a vital skill, enabling us to harness the healing powers of nature and make them available year-round. In this chapter, we delve into the timeless techniques and modern methods of long-term storage and preservation of herbs, ensuring that the bounty of your herbal harvest or purchases remains potent and beneficial for extended periods.

The Imperative of Proper Preservation

The essence of herbal preservation lies in maintaining the integrity and potency of the herbs. The healing properties of plants are highly dependent on how they are stored after harvesting. Incorrect storage can lead to a loss of essential oils, active compounds, and overall efficacy, rendering them less effective or even useless. Therefore, understanding the principles of preservation is crucial.

Understanding the Nature of Herbs

Each herb has unique characteristics - moisture content, essential oil composition, and susceptibility to degradation. Some, like lavender and rosemary, are hardier, while others, such as basil and mint, have higher moisture content and are more prone to spoilage. Recognizing these differences is the first step in determining the best method for preserving each herb.

Drying: The Traditional Method

Drying is perhaps the most ancient and widely used method of preserving herbs. It's a process that requires careful attention to detail to ensure that herbs retain their medicinal qualities.

Optimal Conditions for Drying

Herbs should be dried in a warm, dark, and well-ventilated area. Excessive heat can destroy delicate compounds, while light can lead to fading and loss of potency. A temperature of around 95-100°F (35-38°C) is ideal.

Techniques for Drying

Bundle drying, where herbs are tied together and hung upside down, is effective for many plants.

Screen drying, where herbs are spread out on a mesh screen, is better for plants that may mold if bundled.

Timing is Key

The drying process can take anywhere from a few days to a couple of weeks, depending on the herb and environmental conditions. The herbs are ready when they are crisp and crumble easily.

Freezing: Preserving Freshness

Freezing is an excellent way to preserve the fresh qualities of certain herbs, especially those with high moisture content. The process is simple:

Preparation

Rinse the herbs gently and pat them dry. Chopping them finely or leaving them in larger sprigs is a matter of personal preference.

Freezing Techniques

Herbs can be frozen in a single layer on a baking sheet before being transferred to airtight containers, or they can be frozen in ice cube trays with water or olive oil, perfect for adding to recipes later.

Using Desiccants for Storage

Desiccants like silica gel can be used to maintain dryness in storage containers, especially in humid environments. These materials absorb moisture and protect the herbs from mold and mildew.

Container Preparation

Place a layer of desiccant at the bottom of an airtight container before adding the dried herbs.

Regular Checks

Ensure to check the containers periodically and replace the desiccant if it becomes saturated.

Light and Heat: The Enemies of Herbs

Light and heat can significantly degrade the quality of herbs. Store your dried herbs in a cool, dark place, ideally in airtight containers such as glass jars with tight-fitting lids. Avoid plastic if possible, as it can leach chemicals over time.

Vacuum Sealing for Longevity

Vacuum sealing is a modern method that can greatly extend the shelf life of dried herbs. By removing air, it prevents oxidation and retains the herbs' potency for a longer period.

Labeling: A Crucial Step

Always label your stored herbs with the name and date of storage. It's easy to forget when a herb was harvested or dried, and proper labeling ensures you use the herbs when they are at their best.

Shelf Life Expectations

Dried herbs generally retain their potency for one to three years, depending on the herb and storage conditions. Regularly inspect your stored herbs for any signs of spoilage like mold or a significant decrease in aroma.

Revitalizing Older Herbs

If you find that stored herbs have lost some of their potency, don't be too quick to discard them. Older herbs can be revitalized for use in recipes where the herb's flavor is not the primary focus, such as in broths or stews.

Storing Herbal Preparations

Herbal oils, tinctures, and salves also require careful storage. Tinctures, being alcohol-based, have a longer shelf life and should be stored in dark glass bottles away from light and heat. Oils and salves should be stored in a cool, dark place and used within a year for maximum efficacy.

Embracing Sustainability in Storage

In line with sustainable practices, consider using recycled or reusable containers for storage. This approach not only benefits the environment but also adds a personal touch to your herbal medicine cabinet.

The Joy of Rediscovery

Finally, periodically revisiting your stored herbs can be a journey of rediscovery. It's an opportunity to reconnect with the plants and their properties, reminding us of the cyclical nature of life and the enduring power of nature's gifts.

Through these methods of preservation, we honor the ancient tradition of herbalism, ensuring that the gifts of nature are available to us throughout the year. This chapter not only equips you with practical knowledge but also invites you to partake in the timeless ritual of connecting with the earth and its bounty, a ritual that sustains both our bodies and spirits.

Chapter

11

Chapter 11: The Future of Herbal Medicine

Innovations and research in herbal therapies

The resurgence of interest in herbal remedies is not a mere nod to nostalgia; it is propelled by a growing body of scientific research that validates and expands upon ancient herbal knowledge. This research is uncovering new compounds and mechanisms of action, offering a deeper understanding of how plants exert their therapeutic effects. In this chapter, we will delve into the latest innovations and research in herbal therapies, exploring how they are shaping the future of natural medicine and opening new horizons for holistic health practices.

Revolutionizing Herbal Medicine through Modern Science

At the forefront of this revolution are advancements in biotechnology and phytochemistry. Scientists are now able to analyze plant constituents at a molecular level, unraveling the complex chemistry of herbs. This molecular understanding is crucial, as it allows for the identification of active compounds responsible for a plant's healing properties. For instance, research into the phytochemistry of turmeric has revealed curcumin as a potent anti-inflammatory agent, leading to its widespread use in managing conditions like arthritis and metabolic syndrome.

Another significant breakthrough in herbal medicine research is the use of genomic tools. Nutrigenomics, for example, studies how plant-based compounds interact with our genes. This field is uncovering fascinating insights, such as how certain herbs can modulate gene expression to bolster our immune response or mitigate the effects of stress and aging.

Clinical Trials: Validating Efficacy and Safety

The integration of herbal medicine into modern healthcare is further reinforced by rigorous clinical trials. These trials are essential for validating the efficacy and safety of herbal remedies, ensuring they meet the high standards of contemporary medicine. Clinical trials on herbs like St. John's Wort for depression and Ginkgo Biloba for cognitive enhancement have provided scientific evidence supporting their traditional uses. These studies are crucial for building trust in herbal therapies among both healthcare professionals and the public.

Personalized Herbal Medicine: A New Frontier

Personalized medicine, a rapidly growing field, is also making its way into the herbal realm. This approach tailors treatments to an individual's unique genetic makeup, lifestyle, and health conditions. Personalized herbal medicine could revolutionize how we approach health and disease, moving away from a one-size-fits-all model to more targeted and effective treatments. Imagine a future where herbal remedies are customized based on your genetic profile, ensuring optimal efficacy and minimizing side effects.

Sustainability and Ethical Considerations

As we embrace the potential of herbal medicine, it's imperative to address sustainability. The increasing demand for herbal remedies must be balanced with ethical and sustainable harvesting practices. This not only involves protecting endangered plant species but also ensuring that local communities who have traditionally stewarded these plants benefit from their commercial use. Sustainable cultivation practices are being developed to ensure a steady supply of medicinal herbs without depleting natural resources.

Integrating Technology and Tradition

The future of herbal medicine is also seeing an exciting integration of technology and tradition. Digital tools like apps and online platforms are making herbal knowledge more accessible. These resources provide valuable information on herb identification, preparation methods, and dosage guidelines, making it easier for individuals to incorporate herbal remedies into their daily lives.

Herbal medicine in holistic health practices

As we venture into the future, the role of herbal medicine in holistic health practices presents an intriguing panorama of possibilities and promises. In the realms of personalized healthcare and preventive medicine, herbal remedies offer a unique interplay of tradition and innovation, inviting us to reimagine healthcare in a more integrative, patient-centered manner.

The Harmony of Tradition and Modernity

The resurgence of herbal medicine in modern healthcare is not merely a nod to nostalgia but a response to the growing need for a more comprehensive approach to health and wellness. In this era, where the limitations of conventional medicine become increasingly apparent in dealing with chronic illnesses and lifestyle diseases, the holistic approach of herbal medicine offers a breath of fresh air. It's a practice that doesn't just treat symptoms but looks at the individual as a whole, considering their physical, mental, and emotional health in unison.

Personalized Care: A New Frontier

The concept of personalized medicine is gaining momentum, with a focus on tailoring healthcare to the individual's unique genetic, environmental, and lifestyle factors. Herbal medicine stands at the forefront of this revolution. Imagine a scenario where your healthcare provider not only knows your medical history but also understands your body's specific responses to different herbs. This level of personalization can transform healthcare from a one-size-fits-all model to a more nuanced and effective system.

Preventive Health: The Ancient Wisdom

Preventive health is another area where herbal medicine shines. The philosophy of preventing disease before it occurs aligns perfectly with the principles of many traditional herbal practices. By incorporating herbs into our daily lives, whether through diet, supplements, or topical applications, we actively participate in maintaining our health and preventing future ailments.

The Role of Technology in Herbal Medicine

In this digital age, technology plays a pivotal role in advancing the practice of herbal medicine. With the advent of artificial intelligence and machine learning, we are now able to analyze vast amounts of data on herbal efficacy, safety, and interactions. This technological integration doesn't detract from the authenticity of herbal medicine; rather, it enhances our understanding and application of these ancient remedies.

Community and Sustainability: A Shared Responsibility

Holistic health practices also emphasize the importance of community and sustainability. The ethical harvesting and cultivation of medicinal plants not only ensure the preservation of these precious resources but also foster a sense of connection and responsibility towards our environment. This approach resonates deeply with the ethos of sustainability and environmental stewardship.

The Future: Blending Holistic Practices

Looking ahead, the future of herbal medicine in holistic health practices is bright and promising. We are likely to see a more seamless integration of herbal remedies with other holistic practices such as yoga, meditation, and mindfulness. This integrative approach can provide a more rounded and effective way to manage health and wellness.

Appendices

Glossary of herbal terms

Adaptogen: A class of plants known for helping the body resist stressors of all kinds, whether physical, chemical, or biological. Adaptogens have a normalizing influence on the body, counteracting the adverse effects of stress and promoting homeostasis. Examples include Ashwagandha and Rhodiola.

Alkaloid: A naturally occurring compound found in plants, which typically contains basic nitrogen atoms. Alkaloids have a wide range of pharmacological effects on humans and animals. For instance, caffeine in coffee is an alkaloid.

Anthocyanin: A type of flavonoid, anthocyanin is a pigment that gives many fruits and vegetables their red, purple, and blue colors. Known for their antioxidant properties, anthocyanins are found in berries like elderberry and raspberry.

Aromatherapy: The use of essential oils extracted from plants for healing or soothing purposes. Aromatherapy can be applied through inhalation, topical application, or diffusion. Lavender oil is commonly used for relaxation in aromatherapy.

Bitters: Substances that have a bitter taste, often used to aid digestion. Bitters can stimulate the production of saliva and stomach acids, promoting healthy digestion. Gentian root is a well-known bitter.

Carminative: Herbs that help in relieving gas and bloating in the digestive system. These herbs, such as peppermint and fennel, often have a soothing effect on the gut and can reduce cramping and discomfort.

Decoction: A method of extraction by boiling plant material, especially herbal roots, bark, or seeds, to extract their beneficial properties. A decoction typically involves simmering the plant material for a prolonged period.

Essential Oil: Highly concentrated oils extracted from plants, retaining the natural smell and flavor, or "essence" of their source. Essential oils are used in aromatherapy and various natural remedies.

Flavonoids: A diverse group of plant chemicals (phytonutrients) found in almost all fruits and vegetables. Flavonoids are powerful antioxidants with anti-inflammatory and immune system benefits.

Glycerite: A type of herbal extract where the solvent used is glycerin. Glycerites are a sweet, alcohol-free alternative to tinctures and are particularly suitable for children and those avoiding alcohol.

Herbaceous: Refers to plants that have non-woody stems. They are usually soft-stemmed plants that die back to the ground every year.

Infusion: A very common method of preparing herbs, typically involving steeping leaves or flowers in hot water. Herbal teas are a form of infusion.

Lignan: A type of polyphenol found in plants. Lignans are known for their antioxidant properties and are found in high concentrations in flax seeds and sesame seeds.

Maceration: The process of soaking plant material in cold or room temperature water for an extended period to extract its soluble compounds.

Nervine: Herbs that specifically support the nervous system. Nervines can be stimulant or relaxant. Chamomile and lemon balm are nervines often used for their calming effect.

Oxymel: A traditional herbal preparation made with honey and vinegar. Herbs are infused in this mixture, creating a medicinal syrup. Oxymels are often used for respiratory or digestive issues.

Phenols: Organic compounds found in plants, known for their antioxidant properties. They play an essential role in defending against pathogens and contributing to the plant's color, taste, and smell.

Phytochemicals: Chemical compounds produced by plants, generally to help them thrive or thwart competitors, predators, or pathogens. Many phytochemicals are known for their beneficial effects on human health.

Polysaccharide: A type of carbohydrate that consists of a large number of sugar molecules bonded together. Polysaccharides in herbs, such as those found in Echinacea, are known for their immune-boosting properties.

Resin: A sticky, sap-like substance produced by some plants. Resins often have antimicrobial properties and can be used in healing balms and salves.

Salve: A healing ointment applied to the skin to soothe and heal. Salves are typically made by infusing oils with herbs and then mixing them with beeswax.

Tannins: Naturally occurring compounds found in various plant tissues. Tannins are astringent and can be used for their healing properties on mucous membranes.

Tincture: An extract of a plant or plants, typically made by soaking the plant in alcohol and water.

Tinctures are used for various medicinal purposes and are taken in small doses.

Volatile Oil: Also known as essential oils, these are concentrated plant oils that evaporate easily at normal temperatures. They are responsible for the aroma of many herbs.

Xerophyte: A plant adapted to an arid climate. Xerophytes like sage and lavender have adaptations like reduced leaf area and waxy surfaces to minimize water loss.

Yield (Herbal): The amount of usable plant material obtained after harvesting and processing. Factors like growing conditions and harvesting techniques can affect the yield of medicinal herbs.

Resource guide for further exploration

Deepening Herbal Wisdom through Literature

The world of herbal literature is vast, offering insights into every aspect of plant medicine. For a deeper dive into the science and art of herbalism, consider books like "Medical Herbalism: The Science and Practice of Herbal Medicine" by David Hoffmann, which provides an extensive overview of the subject. For those interested in the intricate relationship between plants and human health, "Adaptogens: Herbs for Strength, Stamina, and Stress Relief" by David Winston and Steven Maimes offers a detailed look at these unique herbs.

Embracing the Digital Age of Herbalism

The internet is a rich resource for herbal enthusiasts. Websites like the American Botanical

Council offer a wealth of information, including access to the HerbalGram journal. For an interactive learning experience, the Herbal Academy provides a range of online courses suitable for beginners to advanced practitioners. Online forums like the HerbMentor community can also be invaluable for connecting with fellow herbal enthusiasts and experts.

Hands-On Learning: Workshops and Schools

Practical experience is key in herbal medicine. The Chestnut School of Herbal Medicine, known for its comprehensive online courses, also offers in-person workshops. For those looking to delve deep, the California School of Herbal Studies provides extensive programs in herbal education, from the basics to advanced clinical training.

Building Community Connections

Local herbalist groups, often found through platforms like Meetup, can be a goldmine of shared knowledge and experience. These groups often organize local herb walks, workshops, and gatherings, offering opportunities to learn from experienced practitioners in a community setting.

Expanding Horizons: Conferences and Seminars

Annual events like the International Herb Symposium bring together herbalists, healthcare practitioners, and educators from around the globe, offering a unique opportunity to learn about the latest research and practices in herbal medicine.

The Joy of Herbal Gardening

For those interested in growing their own medicinal plants, "The Medicinal Herb Grower" by

Richo Cech is a fantastic resource, offering practical advice on cultivating a range of medicinal herbs. Websites like Mountain Rose Herbs not only provide supplies but also offer valuable growing tips and information.

Integrative Health Perspectives

Integrating herbal medicine into modern healthcare requires a balanced approach. "The Integrative Guide to Herbal Medicine" by Sebastian Pole is an excellent resource that bridges the gap between traditional herbal wisdom and contemporary scientific understanding.

Scientific Journals and Research

For a more scientific perspective, journals like the "Journal of Ethnopharmacology" offer peer-reviewed articles on the medicinal properties of plants, providing evidence-based insights into the efficacy of herbal remedies.

Exploring Global Herbal Traditions

The rich tapestry of global herbal traditions can be explored through books like "Healing with Whole Foods: Asian Traditions and Modern Nutrition" by Paul Pitchford, which delves into the intersection of traditional Chinese medicine and modern nutrition.

Legal and ethical considerations in herbal practice

In the realm of herbal medicine, adherence to legal standards is paramount. This is not only a matter of regulatory compliance but also a means of ensuring the safety and well-being of those who turn to these natural remedies for health and healing. Across the United States, laws governing the use of herbal substances vary from state to state, making it crucial for practitioners and enthusiasts alike to be well-versed in the regulations that apply to their specific locations.

For instance, the sale of herbal products is often regulated by the Food and Drug Administration (FDA) under the Dietary Supplement Health and Education Act of 1994 (DSHEA). This act classifies herbal products as dietary supplements, which places them under a different set of regulations compared to pharmaceuticals. It's essential to understand that while these products are not required to be FDA-approved before entering the market, they must be safe for consumption and properly labeled. Mislabeling or making unsubstantiated health claims can lead to severe legal consequences.

Moreover, practitioners who wish to include herbal remedies in their practice need to be aware of the scope of their professional licensure. In some states, specific licensing may be required to practice herbal medicine, especially if it involves diagnosing and treating health conditions. It's a fine line between offering wellness advice and practicing medicine without a license, a distinction that must be clearly understood and respected.

Ethical Harvesting and Sustainability

The ethical considerations in herbal practice extend beyond legal compliance into the realm of sustainability. With the increasing popularity of herbal remedies, the responsibility of ensuring the sustainable use of these natural resources has never been more significant. Ethical harvesting is not just a practice; it's a philosophy that respects and protects the Earth's ecosystems.

Sustainable practices involve understanding the life cycles of plants, recognizing the impact of overharvesting, and knowing when and how to harvest to ensure that plant populations remain robust and healthy. For example, harvesting roots may kill the plant, so it's crucial to do this judiciously and perhaps replant a portion of the root to encourage regrowth. Also, the gathering of wild plants must be done with care, avoiding endangered species and respecting the habitats in which these plants grow.

The Role of Transparency and Accuracy in Information Sharing

Transparency in the dissemination of information about herbal remedies is a cornerstone of ethical practice. Given the vast array of information available, particularly on the internet, ensuring that the advice and information you provide are accurate and based on credible sources is vital. This involves a commitment to continuous learning and staying updated with the latest research in the field of herbal medicine.

Furthermore, it's important to communicate the limitations and potential risks of herbal remedies. While many herbs offer significant health benefits, they may also have side effects or interact with conventional medications. Being open about these aspects helps in building trust and encourages informed decision-making among those seeking herbal treatments.

Respecting Cultural Traditions and Knowledge

Herbal medicine is deeply rooted in various cultural traditions and practices. Respecting these traditions involves recognizing the origins of this knowledge and avoiding the appropriation of practices without proper understanding and acknowledgment. It's crucial to approach herbal medicine with cultural sensitivity and an appreciation for the diversity of practices and beliefs surrounding it.

Acknowledgments

In the creation of "The Lost Herbal Medicine Book," a journey that melded the ancient wisdom of herbal remedies with the practical needs of modern healthcare, the tapestry woven is rich with the contributions of many, each as vital as the deep roots of a centuries-old tree. This endeavor, a blend of traditional knowledge and scientific inquiry, owes its existence to numerous individuals, each bringing their unique essence.

Foremost, my heart swells with gratitude for the herbalists, healers, and wisdom keepers of yore and today. Their unwavering dedication to preserving herbal knowledge lights the path this book treads. From the ancient annals of herbal medicine to the oral traditions echoing through generations, their collective wisdom forms this book's backbone.

A special reverence is reserved for Nonno Renzo, my gruff, shouty grandfather, whose hands, weathered like ancient parchment, first guided mine in the art of picking wild herbs. Those childhood wanderings through the seasons, amidst the symphony of nature, laid the foundation of my herbal journey. Nonno Renzo, with his thunderous voice echoing through the fields and his eyes sparkling with ancestral knowledge, instilled in me the profound respect for nature's gifts. This book is a homage to those early lessons, woven into the fabric of every page.

Immense appreciation goes to modern herbal medicine practitioners who generously lent their insights. Their commitment to marrying tradition with contemporary science has been invaluable, enriching this book with practicality and relevance.

The academic and research community, tirelessly pursuing herbal science's truths, deserves heartfelt thanks. Your studies and papers provided a credibility bridge, linking ancient wisdom and modern understanding.

Crucial, too, were the herbalists and botanists who critiqued early drafts. Your practical perspectives sharpened the book's focus, ensuring accessibility and relevance to our health-conscious, informed female audience.

The local communities and sustainable harvesters, dedicated to ethical gathering practices, inspired Chapter 2's content. Your principles of ethical harvesting and nurturing nature have been guiding beacons.

To my editor, whose finesse and patience transformed the manuscript, I am deeply grateful. Your ability to distill and clarify my thoughts, preserving the core message, has been instrumental.

Acknowledgment is due to the graphic designers and illustrators whose creative talents brought to life the illustrations, making complex information visually appealing and understandable, despite the absence of photographs.

My family and friends' unwavering support has been my anchor, providing motivation and strength. Your belief in this project's importance has been a constant source of inspiration.

To my readers, this book's raison d'être, I extend profound gratitude. Your pursuit of knowledge, commitment to sustainable health, and desire for practical information have been driving forces. May this book empower you to weave herbal remedies into your daily lives, enhancing health and well-being.

Lastly, I acknowledge the project's challenges and learnings. Each hurdle surmounted has been a stepping stone to deeper understanding and growth, much like herbal medicine practice itself – a continuous learning and adaptation process.

About the Author

Ilaria Grandi is a name synonymous with the harmonious blend of traditional herbal wisdom and modern healthcare innovation. As an Italian naturopath specializing in nutrigenetics, immunonutrition, oligotherapy, regenerative phytotherapy, and psychosomatics, Ilaria brings a unique perspective to the world of natural medicine. Her journey into the realm of herbal remedies and natural healing began under the tutelage of her beloved grandfather, Nonno Renzo, whose passion for the natural world was as boundless as the fields and forests where they would forage for wild herbs. This early immersion in nature's bounty sparked a lifelong quest to understand and harness the healing power of plants.

Ilaria's formal education in naturopathy further refined her understanding of the intricate relationship between nature and human health. Her studies led her to explore various facets of natural medicine, with a particular focus on how genetic factors and nutrition influence well-being. This exploration culminated in a specialization in nutrigenetics, where she examines the intersection of genetics, nutrition, and herbal remedies.

Her expertise extends to immunonutrition, where she delves into the role of diet and natural supplements in supporting the immune system. In oligotherapy, Ilaria explores the use of trace elements for therapeutic purposes, while her work in regenerative phytotherapy focuses on using plants to regenerate and heal the body. The field of psychosomatics is another area of her expertise, where she examines the connection between the mind and body, emphasizing the role of mental and emotional well-being in overall health.

Ilaria's approach to natural medicine is characterized by a deep respect for traditional knowledge coupled with a rigorous scientific understanding. This balance is evident in her writings, teachings, and consultations, where she seamlessly integrates ancient herbal practices with contemporary scientific findings. Her work is not just about treating ailments but about empowering individuals to lead healthier, more balanced lives through the understanding and use of natural remedies.

As an established writer and passionate educator, Ilaria's commitment to sharing her knowledge is unwavering. She is known for her engaging, accessible writing style, which reflects her ability to simplify complex concepts into understandable terms. This skill has made her a sought-after author and speaker in the field of natural medicine.

Her latest work, "The Lost Herbal Medicine Book," is a testament to her expertise and dedication. It encapsulates her journey, knowledge, and the wisdom of those who have influenced her, from Nonno Renzo's rustic teachings to the latest advancements in herbal research. Ilaria continues to inspire and educate, driven by her belief in the power of nature and the potential of natural medicine to transform lives.

Printed in Great Britain
by Amazon

38818458R00129